fit + female

fit+female

the perfect fitness and nutrition game plan for your unique body type

geralyn
coopersmith, M.A., C.S.C.S.

WILEY

John Wiley & Sons, Inc.

Published by John Wiley & Sons, Inc., Hoboken, New Jersey
Published simultaneously in Canada

Design and composition by Navta Associates, Inc.

Illustrations by Frank Spinks. Copyright © 2006 by Geralyn Coopersmith

The information contained in this book is not intended to serve as a replacement for professional medical advice. Any use of the information in this book is at the reader's discretion. The author and the publisher specifically disclaim any and all liability arising directly or indirectly from the use or application of any information contained in this book. A health care professional should be consulted regarding your specific situation.

For general information about our other products and services, please contact our Customer Care Department within the United States at (800) 762-2974, outside the United States at (317) 572-3993 or fax (317) 572-4002.

Wiley also publishes its books in a variety of electronic formats. Some content that appears in print may not be available in electronic books. For more information about Wiley products, visit our web site at www.wiley.com.

Library of Congress Cataloging-in-Publication Data:

Coopersmith, Geralyn.
  Fit and female : the perfect fitness and nutrition game plan for your unique body type / Geralyn Coopersmith.
      p. cm.
  Includes bibliographical references and index.
  ISBN-13 978-0-471-73903-6 (paper)
  ISBN-10 0-471-73903-0 (paper)
  1. Reducing exercises. 2. Physical fitness for women. 3. Women—Nutrition.
4. Somatotypes.   I. Title.
  RA781.6.C66 2006
  613.7'1082—dc22

                                                          2005032764

Printed in the United States of America

10 9 8 7 6 5 4 3 2 1

To Logan: You are the light of my life. I love you more than you will ever know.

To Evan: The guy with the blue hair who took my breath away some twenty-three years ago. Thanks for being my partner on this strange and beautiful journey called life.

Contents

Acknowledgments

For my high school yearbook, we were each asked to provide a quote that summarized our philosophy of life. In an effort to distinguish myself from the masses, I chose a quote in French that essentially translated to "the heart is like a suspended lute, those who touch it make it resound." I thought it was a beautiful sentiment—better yet, I thought the fact that it was in French made me look worldly and sophisticated, even though I didn't speak a word of French at the time. (Unfortunately, my best friend, Ilene, took French in college largely because she thought I could help her with her homework. Sorry 'bout that, Bean!)

In writing this acknowledgment, I found that the sentiment behind that quote still rings true with me today. Of all the things in my life that I am grateful for, I am *always* most grateful for the special relationships that sustain me and make "my heart sing." There are so many people who have touched me in some way and contributed to my growth and development that it would take an entire book to list them all, but here goes.

First and foremost, I would like to thank my beautiful family for encouraging me, standing by me, and supporting me through the many months of research and writing that went into this book, especially my son, Logan, and my husband, Evan. Evan, you always believed in this project and in me, and I love you very much for it.

To my mom and dad, Lee and Jerry Coopersmith; my in-laws, Frank Spinks and Laurie Lerner; my sister, Allison Taylor, my brother-in-law, Kent Taylor, and my beautiful nieces, Kaylee Coopersmith, Kendall Rose, Kamryn Grace; my brother and sister-in-law, Bryson and Melissa Coopersmith; and my dearest friend, Ilene Diamond. I am blessed to have all of you in my life. Each of you truly contributed to this dream becoming a reality in your own unique way.

During my sixteen years in this industry, I have been blessed with so many wonderful colleagues who have fostered (and continue to foster) my growth and development that I could write a chapter on that alone. To Melissa Mittman, who started the journey with me as my dear friend and fellow teacher at Marymount. To my Marymount mentors, Dr. Linda Zwiren, Adrienne Jamiel, Haila Strauss, Joan Pagano, and Susan Karp. To my Atrium Club sisters, who remain some of my closest friends today, Jane Bogart and Lori Ende. I think I still have shin splints and hearing loss from teaching all those classes. To the original PT Gang at APEX (Carol, Carolyn, Chris, Donna, Felicia, Greg, Jeff, Jill, Johnny Appleseed, Lippy, Liz, Mark, Mel, Pat, Petey, Paul, Paula, Soo Jin, Susan, and TDB). No matter how far-flung we all are, you will all always be like family to me. Being with you was an amazing work experience that I will never forget. To all of the students I've been honored to teach at Marymount, Hunter College, ACSM, and EFTI. To my Columbia connections, Dr. Ronald DeMeersman, TDB Bach, and Lisa Hoffman.

Right up to today, with all of my Scarsdale Equinox homies. I am so privileged to have a job where I wake up every day and literally can't wait to get to work.

To my many wonderful clients over the years who unwittingly served as human guinea pigs, thanks for entrusting me with your health, letting me share in all the joys of your lives, and always believing in me.

A special shout out goes to the Scarsdale Mastermind Gang (Anthony Renna, Jeff Fields, Les Mebane, Patty Clevenberg, and Raymond Simpson), my current and former partners in crime at Equinox Corporate (Carol Espel, Cheryl Blenk, David Harris, and Joel Greengrass), and, especially, my EFTI teammates, Johanna Subotovsky and Sean Quimby. You are an extraordinary group of individuals who always make me bring my A-Game.

To my dear friend, Joy Bauer of Joy Bauer Nutrition, for encouraging me to write this book. Again, to my father-in-law, Frank Spinks, for sharing his enormous talents by providing the beautiful illustrations found in the book. To my agent, Stacey Glick, at Dystel and Goderich for championing my cause. To the excellent counsel and generosity of my attorney, Ellen Kulka. To Teryn Johnson, Hope Breeman, and Juliet Grames at Wiley for all of your hard work and professionalism. You were all instrumental in making this dream a reality. It's not enough, but thank you, thank you, thank you.

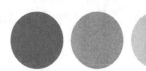

introduction

As an exercise physiologist and a certified personal trainer, I'm proud to have personally helped hundreds of women look and feel their best, by designing diet and exercise programs for individual female body types. For more than fifteen years, I have worked one-on-one with women just like you to create the best fitness game plans for their unique needs.

Many of my clients are new to fitness and are out of shape. When they come to me, they are unhappy with the way their bodies look and feel, but they have no clear plan for how to turn things around. When we first meet, my clients usually tell me that I can't possibly relate to being overweight and out of shape. Whenever I hear that, I have to laugh, because nothing could be further from the truth. The truth is, I know exactly what my clients are feeling because I've been there myself. In fact, that's how I got into this business in the first place.

Been There, Done That ●●●

If you knew me as a kid, you never would have guessed that I'd grow up to be a fitness expert. As a child, I was anything but athletic. Awkward

1

and uncoordinated, I was usually the last (or the near last) to be picked in gym class. I couldn't (and, honestly, still can't) throw or catch a ball. I've always been hopeless with a Frisbee. I have never played on a sports team and have never competed in a major athletic event. Throughout my entire childhood, I consistently shied away from anything physical for fear of making a fool of myself.

During my teen years, between the changes of puberty, my love of sweets, and my hatred of exercise, I became increasingly unhappy with my appearance. I can remember being about fourteen and going on a family vacation. When I put on my bathing suit (for the first time that season) and looked in the mirror, I was horrified by what I saw. I had definitely gained weight over the winter. Gone was the prepubescent body that looked great in a bikini, even on a steady diet of rocky road ice cream and chocolate chip cookies. This body looked completely different. I barely recognized my new shape. I was starting to look like (gasp)—my mom!

I became very depressed at the thought that this was the beginning of the end. I worried that I was on a slippery slope with absolutely no control over my appearance—destined to gain more and more weight, look worse and worse, and hate my body more every day. That's an overwhelming realization when you're only fourteen.

Yet as the years went on, I didn't do anything differently. I continued to eat pretty much as I always had—maybe worse. I had a very negative body image, and I became increasingly self-conscious about my looks.

By my senior year of high school, I was driving a car. That meant freedom to eat when and where I wanted. No longer did I have to eat the slop that they served in the school cafeteria, which meant that I could go to McDonald's whenever I wanted to. And I wanted to—a lot. I went for lunch and sometimes breakfast, too. Egg McMuffins, fries, Quarter Pounders with Cheese, and chocolate shakes were a regular part of my diet.

Although I had never been heavy as a kid, I was gradually becoming a chunky teenager. I can remember being about sixteen and shopping with my sister, Allison. Allison is three years younger than I am and was always naturally skinny and petite. It was back in the early 1980s, and miniskirts were making a comeback. Allison and I were trying some on at the mall with our family. When Allison stepped out of the dressing room, my mom and my grandmother told her how adorable she looked. But when I walked out, my grandmother (who's never been one to mince words) just shook her head as she stared at my legs and said, "Geralyn, you're just too heavy to wear that kind of skirt. You need to have skinny legs and a good figure like your sister." Yikes! As bad as that sounds to a grown woman, believe me, it sounds much worse to an insecure sixteen-year-old! Needless to say, I left that skirt on the hanger. I was so insecure about my looks that I started wearing clothes at least two sizes too big on a regular basis to hide my shape.

About that time, some of my friends told me about a really neat trick. There was a way you could eat whatever you wanted and not gain weight. You simply made yourself throw up afterward, before it turned to fat. That sounded like a perfect solution to me. I actually tried very hard to do it a few times, but, unfortunately (or so I thought at the time), I wasn't able to make myself throw up by putting my finger down my throat.

As my teenage years went on, I became increasingly unhappy with my looks. I looked in the full-length mirror in my closet and analyzed every perceived imperfection of my body. I chastised myself for being fat and lazy, although I was maybe ten or fifteen pounds overweight at most.

I felt out of control with food. I binged on sweets, particularly chocolate, continuing to eat long after I was full. Today, I understand that this behavior was my way of giving myself nurturing and self-love. I was using food to dull pain and frustration that I felt in other areas of my life. At the time, though, I really didn't understand why I was so out of control. Most of this binge eating was done in secrecy, and I felt very guilty and ashamed about it. I had no idea whom to talk to about all of this and didn't know how to turn things around.

My parents' advice on the subject of weight loss was not particularly empowering either. At that point in time, like most people of their generation, my parents believed that gaining weight and getting out of shape were a natural (and inevitable) part of growing older. Whenever I complained to them about my body, they said things like, "This is what happens when you get older" or "You just have a body like Mom's." Neither of which made me feel any better.

After high school graduation, I spent half of the summer on vacation with my family in Israel. By then, I was probably fifteen to twenty pounds overweight and gaining steadily. When we left for the trip, my biggest concern was that this boy I liked would completely forget about me during the month I was gone. My plan was to lose as much weight as I could while I was away, so that he would find me absolutely irresistible when I returned.

In Israel, without a clue as to how to begin, I developed my own fitness "program." It was the first time in my life that I ever cared about being physically active or made a conscious effort to eat well. For someone with no background or education about physical fitness, I actually did some very healthful (and effective) things. I swam in the ocean every day for at least thirty minutes. I drank only water, and I stayed away from desserts and junk food. I ate tons of fresh fruit and vegetables, fish, and chicken. Also, because I wasn't partying with my buddies back home, I wasn't drinking beer or eating greasy late-night diner food. And guess what? The program worked—and fast! I lost more than ten pounds in the five weeks that I was away. I had never looked or felt better in my whole life.

When I returned home, I was tanned, trim, and toned. My friends gave me tons of compliments, and the boy I liked was more attentive than ever. Once I was back in my old routine, though, I fell into the same old habits. By the end of the summer, my weight was climbing again, and when I left for college, one of my girlfriends said, "I really hated you when you got back from Israel; we all did. But I knew you'd gain it all back in no time." I was taken aback. Certainly, it wasn't a very kind thing to say, but, unfortunately, she was right!

As bad as my diet had been in high school, it actually got worse in college! Mostly, I ate breakfast at the mess hall. I loved the breakfasts: bacon, eggs, sausage, buttered toast. But I didn't care for the typical cafeteria fare they served for lunch and dinner, so I usually went to a deli, McDonald's, Burger King, or a pizzeria. I snacked on junk food between meals. I was aware that I was gaining (at least) the "freshman fifteen," but I still did nothing to change my eating habits. It depressed me that all the effort and progress I'd made during the summer was completely undone. I felt totally out of control and increasingly unattractive.

It was around this time that I met my husband, Evan, at college and we started dating. We fell madly in love. Like a lot of teenagers in love, our first few months together were a festival of eating and drinking. We would go to Friendly's, buy a pint of ice cream, and finish it immediately. We'd grab a bucket of KFC every weekend and drink a couple of beers every night. As our love grew, so did our waistlines.

By now, I was at least twenty to twenty-five pounds overweight and continuing to gain. I had never asked Evan directly if he thought I was heavy, because I think I knew what the answer would be. When I finally did work up the nerve to ask, he matter-of-factly said, "Geralyn, you're a beautiful girl, but you could lose ten or fifteen pounds." Yeee-ouch! And as painful as it was to hear, it was true. If anything, he was gilding the lily.

Terrified that I would lose him, I began to diet. I also started taking a movement class at my college a couple of days a week. The class was sort of like modern dance, done for about an hour in bare feet. It was exhausting, a total physical challenge. I left every class completely drenched in perspiration but exhilarated. As a child, I had always loved dancing, but I never thought of it as a form of exercise. I began to think that maybe I was more athletic than I thought. More important, I realized that exercise could actually be fun.

Not only was I working out, I also drastically cut my food intake. I made a vow to eat less than a thousand calories per day, so every night I recorded what I had consumed and chastised myself for anything that put me over the thousand-calorie limit. A typical day's diet consisted of half of a dry bagel and coffee, an apple or a cup of yogurt for lunch, and a Lean Cuisine for dinner. I drank no alcohol, ate no in-between-meal snacks, and allowed myself only a Tootsie Pop or a small Peppermint Patty for dessert.

As my diet became more restrictive, my exercise got more excessive. I decided to work out every day, no matter how I felt. On days when there was no dance class, I did the same kind of routine at home. No rest. No days off. Even when I developed shin splints from overexercising, I ignored them. Eventually, my shin splints became stress fractures, which I ignored as well. I just exercised through the pain as much as I could.

What had started out as a good idea was rapidly turning into an unhealthful obsession. At the time, my sister joked that I knew the exact number of leg lifts needed to burn a leaf of lettuce. The sad truth is, she wasn't far off. I didn't care if I was a little excessive; I was losing weight—and a lot of it!

By the summer after my freshman year, I was the thinnest I had ever been. I had lost about thirty pounds in three months. I could actually fit into my skinny kid sister's size-2 jeans.

Initially, it was great. Everyone complimented me, particularly other women. I figured that if some weight loss was good, more would be better, so, I kept right on losing weight. Before too long, though, words like *skinny* and *amazing* were replaced by words like *emaciated*, *sick*, and *anorexic*.

To me, those words were an exaggeration. I wasn't really that skinny, certainly not as thin as I wanted to be. Maybe I would just drop another ten pounds. I was convinced that people were just saying that because they were jealous of how great I looked—or of my remarkable will-power. It never seriously occurred to me that my diet might be the beginning of an eating disorder until one night when I awoke in a cold sweat from a terrible nightmare. I had dreamed that I was forced to eat birthday cake—on my birthday.

At that point, a rational voice from somewhere deep inside of me acknowledged that I had a problem, but I still wouldn't admit it to anyone else.

One morning shortly after that, my father became frustrated while watching me eat pancakes. Actually, it was just one pancake that I had cut into a million little pieces, and I was chewing each piece for as long as I could. He demanded that I eat that pancake—and a few more. I started to panic. He got angrier and angrier. I was terrified that my dad would force me to start eating more and that I would gain all of my weight back again. We both got pretty irrational, and there was a terrible scene at the breakfast table.

After that, my dad (who's a doctor) was convinced that I needed professional help, so he brought me to the hospital where he is on staff. There I met with a registered dietician named Terri. Terri evaluated my caloric expenditure and my food intake. According to her calculations, I was probably eating at least a thousand calories less than I needed per day. She spoke to me about realistic weight goals, the importance of eating to fuel my active lifestyle, and taking in adequate calcium and iron. The healthy part of me knew what she was saying was true, but I was very frightened of getting fat. Still, I promised her (and my family) that I would try to take her advice by eating more, eating healthfully, and moderating my exercise. Looking back now, I'm very grateful that my Dad got involved at that point. I believe that if not for his intervention, I probably would have descended into a full-fledged battle with anorexia.

Unfortunately, though, my body and food issues still weren't over— far from it. The next several years of my young adulthood were a struggle to maintain some balance. I didn't want to starve myself, but I feared losing control with food and gaining weight. I wanted to eat healthfully, yet not deprive myself of the things I enjoyed. So, I started eating more, but I still really didn't know what I should (or shouldn't) be eating.

I still didn't understand anything about nutrition, although at the time I thought I did. To my mind, a blueberry muffin was a healthful breakfast. Well, I reasoned, it has blueberries in it. I didn't realize that those were actually imitation blueberry bits, along with tons of fat and sugar. For lunch, I would have a burger and fries or some of the greasy pasta offerings at the salad bar. Hey, if it's part of the salad bar, next to the iceberg lettuce, it must be good for you, right? Even dinner, which was probably my most healthful meal of the day, was often greasy Chinese takeout or Mexican food and margaritas.

Occasionally, I noticed that I was gaining weight and went on a diet, which at that time to me meant giving up French fries and existing on fruit salad and cottage cheese. I lost weight and felt good about the weight loss, but I was never sure how to maintain it. My diets always made me feel deprived and resentful that I wasn't able to eat normally. I would lose a few pounds and then be unable to stand the deprivation. Sooner or later, I'd go off the diet and return to my old unhealthful eating habits. It went on this way for several years. I continued to wrestle with the same ten to fifteen pounds. Not a lot of weight, I'll grant you, but enough to make me feel continually frustrated with (and powerless over) my own body.

The one positive thing that happened during those years was that I developed a genuine passion for fitness. I tried new things that I wouldn't have dared to before. I started training with machines and free weights, I took aerobics classes, and I started jogging. I got a natural high from exercise—and I loved the results. I was more toned, fit, and athletic-looking. Most amazing to me, this physical transformation was more than skin deep. Working out made me feel powerful and strong. Best of all, I was working out for myself and not to keep from losing my boyfriend. My workouts became the highlights of my week. The gym became my favorite place to be.

Then when I was twenty-five, I read a book entitled *Do What You Love, the Money Will Follow*, by Marsha Sinetar. I highly recommend this book for people who are at a professional or personal crossroad. The basic principle of the book is that if you love something, you must have passion for it. If you have passion for it, you're probably good at it. In fact, you're probably good enough to make a successful living at it.

I had been working in advertising and public relations up until that time, but I took the message to heart. I decided that I wanted to take a leap and become a full-time fitness professional. With no idea how to get started, I stumbled across a continuing education program in fitness instruction at Marymount Manhattan College. I signed up and started taking the classes. It was truly a life-altering experience. In my year and a half at Marymount, I learned more about the body than I'd ever imagined possible. We took courses in anatomy, kinesiology, exercise physiology, nutrition, and exercise techniques.

The way that I viewed my body, my eating, and my exercising completely changed as a result of this program. I began to consider food the fuel that sustains this miraculous machine known as the human body—food was a friend, not a foe. I started to view exercise as a way to enhance health and well-being, not just tone up flabby thighs or burn off body fat. Most important, the more I learned, the more I realized how much control I actually did have over my weight and my appearance. All of this knowledge made me feel calmer, more in control, and confident about making better choices for myself every day.

Like a convert with a new religion, I became obsessed about sharing this empowering information with girls and women who were struggling with body image issues. I wanted to save others from all of the pain I had dealt with. I wanted to give them the tools that could alter their lives.

In my continual quest for more knowledge, I devoured as much information as I possibly could. Over the next several years, I received six different fitness certifications and eventually went to Columbia University to get my master's degree in exercise physiology. True to the promise of Marsha Sinetar's book, I knew that I had found my life's calling. Within a very short period of time, my career skyrocketed.

New and wonderful opportunities seemed to lie around every corner. Shortly after I graduated from Marymount, I was asked to join its faculty. *New York* magazine selected me as one of the "Trainers to Watch." I joined and then became the associate fitness director at what was then one of New York's most exclusive fitness clubs, APEX. I appeared in numerous magazines: *Elle, Glamour, Mademoiselle, Weight Watchers, Fit Pregnancy, Marie Claire, Family Circle, Seventeen, Cosmopolitan*, and *Redbook*. I was asked to be the resident fitness expert on a new television show, *Prevention Magazine's BodySense*. I did a few commercials and appeared in various TV news segments. Currently, I am the fitness expert on *Simplify Your Life*, now entering its third season on the Fine Living Channel (www.fineliving.com). I was also the fitness consultant for a number of books, including *The Complete Idiot's Guide to Total Nutrition*, *Jay Walking*, and *The Runner's World Guide to Pregnancy*.

Today, I work for Equinox Fitness, which I believe (and I think most people in the industry would agree) is far and away the finest chain of health clubs in the nation. I am privileged to be the senior manager of the Equinox Fitness Training Institute (EFTI). Together with Sean Quimby and Johanna Subotovsky, I design and implement the educational programs for all of the trainers in our thirty-one clubs, or more than eight hundred personal trainers nationwide. Truly, I am living my dream. I am blessed to have a job where I jump out of bed each day, excited to come to work.

The industry has been very good to me, but, honestly, I attribute my success not to my education but rather to my passion for what I do. I genuinely care about my clients, particularly my female clients. More than anything, I want to empower women with the knowledge and the tools they need to have bodies they love—and to love the bodies they have.

I believe that my programs have been effective for several reasons. For one thing, I take into consideration the specific needs and challenges of individual female body types. Does my client gain weight easily? Where does she store excess body fat? Around the middle or on her hips and thighs? Does she tend to gain muscle mass easily? All of these are factors I must consider when designing a wellness plan that ensures results. As a wife and a mother with a full-time career, I understand that in order to be effective, fitness must fit into a busy woman's life, not the other way around.

Finally, I always try to make staying in shape fun. Nobody's going to keep doing something in the long run if she doesn't get some enjoyment from it. Working out and eating right should be two things that you do purely for yourself, because you love yourself and want to feel (and look) as good as possible.

I designed this book to share with you everything I've learned about fitness. I want to give you the tools you'll need to transform yourself into the best that you can be. Changing your body isn't just about improved health, physical attractiveness, and self-confidence. Certainly, these are all great benefits, but, more important, changing your physical body is a powerful metaphor for your ability to make major changes in other areas of your life as well. Every time you look into the mirror and see your new body, you are reminded that you made this happen. It's proof that by putting your mind to something and taking daily actions toward achieving your goals, you really can turn dreams into realities!

I feel privileged that you have put your trust in me to guide you on this wonderful journey. So, with that in mind, let's begin.

what we *want* to look like—and why

An Epidemic of Self-Hatred ●●●

Maggie

Most women would kill to look like Maggie. Arguably the most fit woman in the gym, Maggie is a runner, a biker, and a serious weight lifter. At five feet three inches, she weighs about 100 pounds, has 12 percent body fat, and is pretty and petite. She has amazing definition in her torso, a small round bottom, and sinewy, well-defined arms. It's hard to believe she's a mom in her early forties. She is a true athlete, capable of doing virtually anything I throw at her.

To look at her, no one would imagine that Maggie actually hates her body. As her personal trainer, though, I know the truth. During our training sessions, she constantly complains about her "fat thighs" and her "lard ass." At first, I thought these statements were Maggie's way of fishing for compliments, but over time I realized that she was actually serious. In fact, Maggie is so dissatisfied with her appearance that she recently decided to have liposuction on her legs.

When she told me this in confidence, I was dumbfounded. For the life of me, I couldn't imagine: (1) what kind of doctor would agree to do this procedure on someone who looks like her, and (2) where the heck he plans on sucking out the fat from!!—there's nothing there that I can see.

It's moments like this where, as a fitness professional, I feel as if I live in a world gone mad. Here is this beautifully toned creature, yet no amount of evidence can convince her that she has a fabulous body.

Unfortunately, Maggie is not alone. Not by a long shot. Sadly, there is a virtual epidemic of female body bashing in this country. We live in a society where most women are unhappy with the bodies they have—regardless of what they look like. In fact, in one study, a unbelievable 90 percent of the women surveyed said they were dissatisfied with their appearance.

Consider these other sobering statistics:

75 percent of normal-weight women think they are overweight.

90 percent of women overestimate their body size.

70 percent of women between the ages of thirty and seventy said that they wished they were thinner.

Seven out of ten U.S. women are "on a diet" at any given time.

89 percent of all plastic surgery is performed on women.

No wonder the diet industry generates a staggering $50 billion annually! Perhaps most disturbing of all—despite this amount of money spent on weight loss—47 million women in this country are currently overweight, and diet failure rates are as high as 95 percent!

The Culture of Unhappiness ●●●

The Barbie Body

Why are so many women so unhappy with their bodies? Why are so many of us trying to change ourselves?

After fifteen years as a certified personal trainer and an exercise physiologist, I can tell you that one of the main reasons that women are disappointed by their appearance is that they have a distorted concept of what a healthy, "normal" female body is supposed to look like in the first place.

Every day, I meet with female clients to discuss their fitness goals. Almost all of the women I speak to tell me that they are working out not for the many health benefits but rather to alter something about their appearance. Whenever I ask specifically what it is that my client would like to change about her body, invariably she begins to describe the "Barbie Body." She tells me that she wants to be longer, leaner, with thin legs, a small waist, and large, buoyant breasts. In fact, I have never had a client say that she wanted to be shorter, bulkier, with thick legs and a round middle and small (or saggy) breasts. It's just not the ideal that most of us have internalized.

Nearly every woman I have ever met wants to look like an unnatural (and virtually unattainable) standard, a standard that most of us have internalized to the point that we believe it to be a desirable and realistic goal. In other words, the person most women believe they should strive to be is usually someone they could never realistically expect to become. Like it or not, though, the Barbie Body is a part of our collective female psyche.

Most of us grew up with Barbie. We changed her outfits and marveled at her perfect blond hair, her large nippleless breasts, her inconceivably small waist, and, of course, those long, long legs. Barbie has no body fat, no lumps, no bumps, no bulges, no unsightly veins—she is pure plastic perfection. We began to believe (either consciously or subconsciously) that this was what we would look like when we became women.

However, normal female physiology being what it is, most of us ended up looking dramatically different than Barbie. In other words, we ended up looking like, well—real women. We developed normal body fat on our legs, thighs, and/or tummies. Our legs were too short, our breasts weren't big enough—or perhaps they were too big. Bottom line, no matter how puberty affected our bodies, it's a safe bet that we didn't magically transform into the Barbie doll that we always thought we would become. Over time, because of the chasm between our fantasy and our reality, most of us began to feel increasingly frustrated with our appearance and even hostile toward the bodies that we inhabit.

Certainly, on a logical level, most women understand that Barbie's anatomy has little to do with reality. Just look around. There isn't a whole lot of real-world evidence for the notion that women actually do look like Barbie. Yet on a deeper level, most of us, in our heart of hearts, still yearn to look that way. There's slim chance of that.

The fact is, Barbie's dimensions have so little to do with reality that a woman would have just as much chance of turning into Tinkerbell, Minnie Mouse, or Betty Boop. Consider the following statistics:

If Barbie were a flesh-and-blood woman, she would be at least five feet nine inches and would weigh only 110 pounds.

According to the Met Life Ideal Height and Weight Tables, the normal weight range for a five-foot, nine-inch woman is actually 129 to 170 pounds.

The Met Life Ideal Height and Weight Tables list 110 pounds as an appropriate weight for a small-framed woman under five feet two inches.

The average American woman is actually five feet four inches tall and weighs 140 pounds.

If Barbie were a real person, her bust-waist-hip measurements would be 39-18-33.

The average American woman's measurements are 35-28-38.

In a recent study, a group of scientists created a computer-generated model of a woman with Barbie-doll proportions. According to their analysis, based on those proportions, Barbie's back would be too weak to support the weight of her upper body. Moreover, a torso of that size would be too narrow to contain more than half of a liver and a few centimeters of bowel. Their conclusion: an individual with Barbie's dimensions would likely suffer from chronic diarrhea—and would ultimately die from malnutrition. Not a very pretty picture at all.

Yet for most of us, the Barbie Body still represents the gold standard of womanly beauty. It is a lie that most women believe (on some deeper level) to be a truth—a form of collective insanity. Unfortunately, the vast chasm between this deep-seated belief and reality sets women up for a lifetime of body hatred and self-loathing.

Models: Normal Women or Freaks of Nature? ●●●

Unfortunately, our unrealistic role models didn't stop with Barbie. As we moved through puberty and into our teens, our icons of female perfection shifted from the Barbie dolls that we played with to the real-life "dolls" who graced billboards and the pages of fashion magazines—models.

Nearly everywhere we turn, we are inundated with photos of air-brushed female perfection. Images of models are so prevalent in our daily lives that it's easy to believe that this is what real women are supposed to look like. It's not. Although models are flesh-and-blood people, their dimensions have about as much to do with normal human female bodies as Barbie's do. Think about it. The very reason that models are paid thousands of dollars per day for people to take photographs of them is that they have highly unusual looks. Specifically they are (1) more attractive than the average woman, (2) taller than the average woman, and (3) much thinner than the average women. In other words, they represent an unusual exception to the rule, not the rule itself—and not necessarily the ideal. We need to put models in an appropriate context and appreciate them for being the beautiful freaks of nature that they are. Consider:

The average model is actually thinner than 98 percent of American women.

Only 5 percent of the women on the entire planet have a model's body type naturally.

The average model wears a size 2 to 4.

The average American woman wears a size 12 to 14.

The average model is five feet eleven inches and weighs 110 pounds.

The average woman is five feet five inches and weighs 145 pounds.

According to the Met Life Height and Weight Tables, the normal weight range for a five-foot, eleven-inch woman is actually between 135 and 176 pounds.

Putting it another way, most women aren't five feet eleven inches—and even those who are, aren't supposed to weigh 110 pounds! Based on those proportions, the average model is actually *thinner* than a Barbie doll!

Yet on some level, most of the women I meet still believe that if they work hard enough at it, diet enough, work out enough, and get the right plastic surgeon, they, too, can look like a supermodel. The reality is, the overwhelming majority of us do not, cannot, and should not even try to look like fashion models.

All of which begs the question: if models' bodies are so unrealistic, why don't advertisers use more realistic role models instead?

There are several reasons for this. For one thing, a model's straight-up-and-down figure doesn't compete with the clothing. This allows the clothing to hang unobstructed by hips or breasts, as if on a living clothes hanger.

Also, because the camera provides only a two-dimensional image, it flattens out the body, adding at least ten pounds to a woman's appearance. That means someone needs to be remarkably slight in real life to still appear slender on film. In fact, models who are sometimes shockingly thin in real life often don't appear to be emaciated in photographs or on TV.

Even the standards for what a fashion model is supposed to look like have gotten progressively thinner over the last thirty years. Back in 1968, the average model was 8 percent thinner than the average American woman. Today's average model is about 23 percent thinner than the average American woman.

Finally, and most significantly, it is in the advertisers' best interest to perpetuate a culture in which women hate their own bodies. Think about it. Women who are unhappy with their bodies make great consumers. The stronger a woman's drive to transform herself into something (which in reality she has no chance of becoming), the more motivated she will be to buy various products. The media constantly deliver subtle messages reminding women that they are inherently flawed and don't measure up to the standard. Marketers play on this insecurity by implying that if women purchase a particular product, they will be "fixed." Scores of products, from exercise equipment to face creams, are advertised this way.

Perhaps the greatest irony of all is that these beautiful models whom most of us are striving to look like don't actually look like this either!

We often forget that advertisers spend thousands and thousands of dollars just to get a single flawless image. Thanks to the work of makeup experts, hairdressers, stylists, photographers, lighting experts, and airbrush artists, these already "perfect" women have been made to appear even more so. With new advances in digital retouching, nearly every woman in print ads today is basically a painting, altered in every imaginable way to be even more flawless than she already is. No wrinkles, no cellulite, no blemishes, and thighs as thin as the art director wants. No wonder most of us are disappointed when we look in the mirror and see something very different from the ads in magazines!

Research suggests that the more exposure that women or girls have to unrealistic body images in magazines and on TV, the greater their levels of body-image dissatisfaction. Strong societal pressures on females to be flawless begin at an age far younger than most of us realize.

An estimated 50 percent of thirteen-year-old girls say that they are unhappy with their appearance. By the age of eighteen years, that number increases to a whopping 80 percent! In 1970, the average age at which a girl started dieting was fourteen; by 1990, the average age had dropped to eight. In a survey of the readers of *Teen People* magazine, nearly 70 percent of the girls surveyed said that models in magazines influenced their idea of the perfect body shape. Twenty-seven percent of the teenage girls polled said that they felt pressured by the media to have a perfect body. Middle and high school girls who read fashion magazines frequently are twice as likely to have dieted and three times as likely to have started working out to lose weight, as compared to less frequent readers. Here are some more disturbing findings:

Girls as young as five have expressed fears about getting fat.

A study of ten-year-olds revealed that 80 percent of them were afraid of being overweight.

In one study, 51 percent of nine- and ten-year-old girls said that they felt better about themselves if they were "on a diet."

The number-one wish for girls ages eleven to seventeen is to "be thinner."

In one survey, some of the primary school girls interviewed actually said that they would prefer to live through a nuclear holocaust, lose both of their parents, or get sick with cancer rather than be fat.

Despite what you might expect, it's not just girls and young women who obsess about their looks. Studies suggest that older women feel as much pressure to be thin as their younger counterparts do. A survey of women ages thirty to seventy-four found that 70 percent of them were discontented with their weight—even though all of the women surveyed were of normal weight! In fact, some studies suggest that women between the ages of forty and fifty-five are actually the group least happy with their figures. Elderly women (defined as older than sixty-six years of age) have body-image dissatisfaction similar to that of younger women, but they are less likely to take actions to change their appearance.

Clearly, there is an epidemic of female self-hatred in this country. Whether women are overweight or not, young or old, the majority are unhappy with their own bodies. And as long as women compare themselves to unnatural standards, this trend is likely to continue. As women, we need to constantly remind ourselves that the images presented in the media have little or nothing to do with reality. We need to look around in the everyday world and remind ourselves what women actually look like.

Look at your mother, grandmother, sisters, friends, and coworkers. How many of them are flawless? Yet don't you find something beautiful about almost every one, once you get to know her? Pretty eyes, nice skin, silky hair. Sure, we all look a bit different from one another. We all have our imperfections and our own particular brand of beauty. None of us is flawless. Just like snowflakes, all of us are remarkable and no two of us are alike.

So, if as a sex we aren't meant to look anything like the images presented in the media, what are we supposed to look like? In the next chapter, we'll examine the reality of what the female form actually is and explore the notion of reasonable, attainable goals for looking our best.

what we *do* look like—and why

In a gym where I worked a few years ago, there was a member who wanted to be a personal trainer. We'll call her Sue. Unfortunately, Sue had no formal education or training. Worse yet, she was a compulsive overexerciser and an anorexic.

No matter the time of day, Sue was always at the gym working out. She was shockingly thin, her workout tights literally hung off her body, her hair was dry and lifeless, and a fine layer of lanugo (a downy hair associated with anorexia) covered all of her exposed skin.

Most of the guys in the gym found her "gross" and "creepy looking," but I was stunned by the number of women who told me that they thought she looked "amazing" and had a "great body." More disturbingly, when she announced that she was accepting personal training clients, the number of women who came running to sign up with her was staggering.

For me, this was proof that a woman's notion of what the ideal female body is supposed to look like is fundamentally different from a man's. The fact is, most of us hate the very things that make us women. We bemoan the size of our breasts, our thighs, our hips, and our buttocks. Ironically, these are the exact body parts that make men salivate. Yet the kind of body that most of my female clients long for is one with virtually no hips, no buttocks, no belly, and long, extremely thin legs, but large, perky breasts.

For better or worse, the chances of having such a body naturally are slim to none. Show me a very slender woman with virtually no curves but large, buoyant boobs, and most of the time I'll show you

> A woman with freakish genetics (about 5 percent of the world's population)
>
> A woman with an eating disorder—and implants
>
> A woman who has had liposuction—and implants

As women, we are supposed to have curves. We are biologically designed to have more body fat than our male counterparts—or than prepubescent girls. Body fat is one of the things that makes us female in the truest sense of the word.

If not for our body fat, we wouldn't be able to get pregnant, give birth, or breastfeed. I think most women who've had kids would agree that these are some of the most miraculous experiences of the female life cycle. Fat is one of the substances that makes these life-altering events possible—a necessary trade-off in the equation. The trick with body fat is having enough for good health and not so much that it becomes a health concern.

Having too little body fat can result in menstrual dysfunctions, musculoskeletal problems, and osteoporosis. Having too much fat is associated with high blood pressure, high cholesterol, type 2 diabetes, and even female cancers.

Actually, the body is supposed to have two kinds of fat: essential body fat and storage body fat. Essential body fat is just that, fat required by the body for survival. This type of fat is found in the spinal cord, the brain, the heart, the lungs, the liver, the mammary glands, and the uterus. In women, this essential fat represents about 12 percent of the body's weight.

What most women fail to understand, however, is that in addition to our essential fat, we also need a certain percentage of storage or nonessential fat. Storage fat is important because it provides cushioning for the body and the internal organs, provides insulation from the cold, and gives us storage energy.

Some of us have more body fat, others have less, but every woman has a place (or several places) in which her body tends to hold body fat. It may be in the belly area (the apples) or on the hips, the buttocks and the thighs (the pears), but the vast majority of us have at least some visible body fat somewhere.

Unfortunately, these are usually the body parts that women hate. They see the body fat, obsess about it, and wish that it wasn't there. Most women refuse to accept that to a certain extent, it's supposed to be there.

Everything You Wanted to Know about Cellulite but Were Afraid to Ask ●●●

Cellulite is just body fat, plain and simple. Because of its location, though (right underneath the epidermis, the uppermost layer of the skin), cellulite has a distinctive appearance. The fat in these areas is packed into little chambers of skin and connective tissue, causing it to bunch up and push against the skin's surface and creating a dimpled or orange peel–like appearance. Cellulite is more of a concern for women than for men, because men have a thicker epidermis layer than women do. It's most commonly seen on the thighs, the buttocks, the lower abdomen, and the backs of the upper arms.

Cellulite can actually be categorized in two ways. The first is compression cellulite, which is caused by briefly pushing fat cells against the skin's surface during a temporary change in body position. This type of cellulite is sometimes seen when a woman sits down in a short skirt and crosses her legs.

The second type of cellulite is consistent feature cellulite. In this form, body fat with a mattresslike appearance can be seen in a given area all the time, regardless of the body position.

Here are some other interesting facts about cellulite:

> Cellulite's appearance is largely a function of variations in the skin's structure, which makes some women more predisposed to having it based simply on their genetics.

Variations in skin structure between men and women are largely due to differences in hormones. Men with fewer male hormones are more likely to have cellulite.

Because cellulite has to do mostly with skin formation, it is often seen even in very slender women. However, its appearance is usually exaggerated in overweight women.

Women with greater muscular development tend to have less visible cellulite than women with less development. Female athletes consistently have less cellulite than their non-athletic counterparts do.

Changes in the skin's elasticity due to age and even crash dieting often increase the appearance of cellulite.

Liposuction is not very successful in altering the appearance of cellulite and can sometimes actually worsen it.

So now for the million-dollar question: What (if anything) can be done about cellulite?

Unfortunately, avoiding cellulite (or reducing its appearance) is not a function of any single thing. There is no one specific exercise that will burn or sculpt cellulite off any particular body part. A woman can do several things, however, to reduce its appearance. These include

Lowering her overall body fat by following a healthful diet that doesn't contain more calories than she needs.

Doing cardiovascular (aerobic) exercise, consistently, three to five times per week for twenty to sixty minutes each time.

Performing regular resistance exercises, two to three times per week, to tone the legs. If the body fat underneath the skin's surface is resting on flaccid muscle tissue, this worsens the fat's appearance.

How Much Fat Are We Supposed to Have? ●●●

So, the question remains: How much body fat is enough? How much is too much? Experts agree that women need at least 12 to 14 percent essential body fat just to sustain vital bodily functions such as menstruation. What many women fail to realize is that we need at least 2 to 4 percent body fat beyond that for optimal health and wellness.

On the other end of the spectrum, having more than 32 percent body fat raises your risks for developing serious health problems, such as high blood pressure, cancers (of the breasts, the uterus, the kidneys, and the colon), gallbladder disease, coronary artery disease, diabetes, and osteoarthritis.

Therefore, most experts recommend that body fat percentages for normal, healthy women should be in the 18 to 25 percent range.

The following chart shows classifications of various body fat ranges for women.

Body Fat Ranges

Athletic	<17%
Lean	17–22%
Normal	22–25%
Above Average	25–29%
Overfat	29–35%
Obese	35+%

In addition, other factors determine the appropriate body fat percentages for a given population. They include

Sex. Women are supposed to have more fat than men have.

Age. Older people usually have more fat than their younger counterparts do, which is a result of the loss of muscle tissue and an increase in body fat typically associated with the aging process.

Activity Level. Athletes typically have less fat than nonathletes do, which in some sports (such as track) gives them an advantage.

Heredity. Some individuals are just naturally more prone to gain and hold onto body fat than others are.

The Scale ●●●

Ironically, the method that most of us use to monitor our weight—the scale—actually gives us the least amount of information about what that weight consists of. In other words, you could be light on the scale but have a relatively high percentage of body fat. Or you could be relatively heavy on the scale but actually be quite lean.

In this culture, we have a tendency to take the information that we get from any device (such as a scale) very literally. In other words, "the scale says that I weigh 152 pounds," so it must be true. Well, maybe it is—and maybe it isn't.

The fact is, the numbers that you see on a scale can be affected by many factors, including your menstrual cycle, your hydration status, your sodium intake, your eating, your exercising, and more.

To illustrate just how widely scale numbers can vary, let's look at twenty-four hours in "The Life of the Scale," using my client Alexa as an example.

> 6:30 A.M.—Alexa gets up and gets on the scale. She weighs 133 pounds undressed, after emptying her bladder.

> 7:30 A.M.—Alexa steps on the scale wearing her bathrobe, after eating breakfast and drinking two cups of coffee. Her weight is now 135.5 pounds.

> 10:30 P.M.—Alexa steps on the scale naked, before putting on her PJs. She went out to dinner and had Chinese food and two glasses of wine. Her weight is now 138 pounds!!!

What do you think the odds are that Alexa gained five pounds—in a single day? Slim to none, right?

Yet many women take scale weight to be the gospel truth! I cannot tell you how many times clients have said to me, "I gained three pounds yesterday."

Think about that for a minute. To gain one pound, you need to eat 3,500 calories over and above what your body requires to maintain itself and provide you with adequate energy. That means to gain three pounds, you would have to eat three times that much, or 10,500 calories over and above what your body needs. So, unless you spent your day as an entrant in a pie-eating contest, it's highly unlikely that you gained three pounds in a single day!

Just a pint of water (which has zero calories) weighs a pound on the scale. In fact, sometimes after a high-intensity workout, clients have said to me, "What a great workout—I just lost two pounds!" Of course, they didn't really lose two pounds of body fat; they just sweated out the equivalent of two pounds of water. And that water loss needs to be replaced immediately to avoid dangerous health consequences such as heat illness.

Seeing those numbers fluctuate on daily basis really terrorizes my female clients. Worse yet, some women insist on stepping on the scale several times per day! Talk about making yourself crazy!

This is the reason I recommend that people weigh themselves only one time per week, at most. Ideally, these weigh-ins should be done buck naked on a Wednesday morning after going to the bathroom and before you eat or drink anything.

Why Wednesdays? Well, for one thing, most of us go a little crazy on the weekends. We tend to overindulge a bit. Moreover, the types of foods that we go overboard with typically have a higher sodium content, which can make us retain water. Because Wednesday is smack-dab in the middle of the weekdays, the effects of those little pig-outs should be much less.

So, if the scale isn't the best way to keep tabs on one's percentage of body fat, what is? Let's look at some more effective (and less effective) ways to measure body fat.

Hydrostatic Weighing

The gold standard for measuring body composition is called hydrostatic weighing. This is a process in which someone gets dunked into a large tank of water, and the density of the body is measured by the amount of water that is displaced, or splashed out. The more dense (or lean) the individual is, the more water that person will displace.

The idea is similar to tossing a giant rock into an overfilled bucket of water or tossing a sponge of the same size into the same type of bucket. The rock will sink to the bottom of the bucket and splash out more water, whereas the sponge will float on the surface, displacing little or none. The more muscular the person, the denser she will be, and the more she will sink and displace water. That's why this method is also called densitometry. The obvious problem, of course, is that unless you happen to have a giant hydrostatic tank in your living room (I had to get rid of mine because it clashed with the couch), it isn't very practical.

Skinfold Measurements

The next-best method, after hydrostatic weighing, is skinfold measurements. This technique involves measuring the thickness of the skin at particular sites using a special device known as a caliper. This method makes use of the knowledge that more than 50 percent of the body's fat is stored underneath the skin. By taking measurements and entering them into a specific formula, a trained professional can give a reading that is probably within 3 to 4 percent of a hydrostatic measurement. Although very few people could make use of this method at home, most health clubs usually have at least one person on their staff who is trained at using skinfold calipers. This method is best repeated every few months because (for better or worse) it isn't very sensitive to day-to-day fluctuations.

Bioelectrical Impedance Analysis

Bioelectrical impedance analysis (BIA) is another method that has risen in popularity over the last few years due to the increase in hand-held bioelectrical impedance machines and specialized body fat scales.

The concept behind bioelectrical impedance machines is a simple one. These devices send a small electrical current from one end of the body to the other (hand to hand or foot to foot). The time that it takes for the current to travel from point A to point B is measured. In general, current will move faster through lean body tissue than through fat tissue. Faster transmission should mean a leaner individual.

The problem with BIA is that there are many ways to get a false reading. Even under the best of circumstances, a whole host of conditions needs to be met for these readings to be accurate. Incidentally, most of the people who use these machines in their homes probably aren't aware of these requirements. Here's a partial list of what you need to do to have an accurate BIA reading:

Don't eat or drink within four hours of the test.

Don't exercise within twelve hours of the test.

Be sure to empty your bladder completely before testing.

Don't consume alcohol within forty-eight hours of the test.

Worst of all, BIA tends to dramatically overestimate the body fat of lean individuals and underestimate the body fat of heavier people. That's why, when asked by my clients whether I prefer a plain old bathroom scale to a fancy scale with BIA, I'll take the simple bathroom scale every time. Even though the number on the scale doesn't tell the entire story, scales with BIA can make you even crazier by giving you two potentially flawed readings at once.

Body Mass Index

The body mass index is a calculation that relates a person's weight to his or her height. The BMI is widely used today; the National Institutes of Health (NIH) currently favors the BMI instead of traditional height/weight tables.

Yet the BMI also has drawbacks. For a sedentary individual, the BMI is a good indicator of the amount of total body fat that the person has. For anyone who works out regularly (and therefore has more muscle tissue), however, the BMI overestimates the amount of body fat the person has because it assumes most of the weight to be fat. The BMI is also less accurate for young adults who are not fully grown, adults who are naturally very lean, and adults over sixty-five years of age.

$$ \text{BMI} = \left(\frac{\text{Weight in pounds}}{(\text{Height in inches}) \times (\text{Height in inches})} \right) \times 703 $$

The National Institutes of Health defines "overweight" as having a BMI of 27.3 or more for women and 27.8 or more for men. Obesity is defined as a BMI of 30 or more, which usually translates into being about 30 pounds overweight.

BMI Ranges

Adults	Women	Men
Anorexia	<17.5	
Underweight	<19.1	<20.7
Normal range	19.1–25.8	20.7–26.4
Marginally overweight	25.8–27.3	26.4–27.8
Overweight	27.3–32.3	27.8–31.1
Very overweight or obese	>32.3	>31.1
Severely obese	35–40	
Morbidly obese	40–50	
Super obese	50–60	

Waist-to-Hip Ratio

A great deal of research supports the notion that people with apple-shaped bodies are at greater risk of developing major health problems than are those with pear-shaped figures. The waist-to-hip ratio can provide a quick snapshot of (1) how you store body fat, and (2) whether you are at risk for weight-related health problems.

To calculate your waist-to-hip ratio, simply measure the narrowest circumference of your waist and the circumference of your hips at the widest part of your buttocks with a tape measure, then divide the waist measurement by the hip measurement.

Women should have a ratio of .80 or less. Men should have a ratio of less than 1.0. The higher the number, the more apple-shaped the individual and the greater his or her risk of developing weight-related health problems such as heart disease and type 2 diabetes.

Lean, Not Skinny ●●●

Keep in mind that being thin simply means that a woman has less total body weight, but that isn't necessarily a good thing. Being skinny does not mean you are toned, free of cellulite, fit, or (most important) healthy.

When most women step on the scales, they hope to see as small a number as possible. Usually, they don't care what that weight consists of—fat, muscle, or water—just as long as there isn't a lot of it! But they should care.

Rather than focusing on their weight and trying to weigh less and less, women should focus on the quality of that weight—their body composition. In the long run, it's better for women to be leaner rather than skinnier.

What's the difference?

A skinny woman typically

Has little or poor muscle tone

Develops stooped or poor posture from lack of strength in the upper back and the shoulders

Has a greater chance of gaining weight as she ages due to being undermuscled

Has an increased risk of developing osteoporosis she grows older

Whereas a lean woman typically

Looks fit and trim

Has good muscle tone

Has good posture, which improves her appearance and keeps her looking younger, longer

Is more metabolically active, and therefore has less chance of gaining weight in the long run

Has greater protection against musculoskeletal problems and osteoporosis

Slow Down, You're Losing Too Fast! ●●●

When we lose weight, we shouldn't do it in a way that will make us more likely to gain again in the future. When most women go on a diet, they want to lose as much weight as they can, as quickly as possible. Despite what diet advertisements would like you to believe, though, it actually *is* possible to lose too much weight too fast.

The body will only let go of so much body fat at one time. Research suggests that when people lose more than two pounds per week (so-called crash dieting), they also lose significant amounts of lean body tissue in the process.

When I say this to my clients, the usual response is, "So what?" Most women don't really care if they sacrifice a few pounds of muscle in the weight-loss process. They usually remind me that they don't want to develop big muscles anyway.

The only problem with this line of logic is that for every pound of muscle tissue we lose from dieting, we end up burning approximately *30 to 50 fewer calories per day*. In other words, lose 3 or 4 pounds of lean body tissue and we burn as many as 200 fewer calories each day—or about 1,400 fewer calories in a week. That represents a possibility of gaining almost half a pound per week from eating exactly the same as we did before!

Therefore, rather than just caring about having a low number on the scale, women should focus on being leaner—even if sometimes this might mean they end up being heavier on the scale than they think they should be.

In the next chapter, we'll look at how women get out of shape in the first place and what new behaviors and attitudes we can develop to prevent this from happening in the future.

the secrets of female fitness: how we get fat, how we stay fit

Running on Empty ● ● ●

Women amaze me. As a gender, we have a seemingly endless capacity to anticipate and attend to the needs of others. Most of the women I know have at least two full-time jobs, as managers of their families and as workers outside the home. Some have their own businesses, some work for others, others are committed to volunteer work, but all of them have a staggering amount of responsibility. The downside of all this giving is that something else has to give. Too often, for many of the women I know, that something is the quality of their own lives.

As women, we are all too willing to sacrifice the quality of our day-to-day existence for our kids, our partners, our jobs—all those people and things that we truly value. When schedules get hectic, we have an incredible ability to run on fumes, with too little sleep, haphazard eating habits, and catch-as-catch-can downtime. Sooner or later, however, all of this self-neglect does reach a threshold. We wake up one day and find that we are exhausted, out of shape, and just plain burned-out.

Often we are disgusted with the way we look and feel. Worst of all, we feel locked in a cycle of doing for others, with no way out. But there is an escape hatch out of this unresourceful state. We must immediately start giving to ourselves.

Putting Yourself First ●●●

The truth is, you can't be a nurturer to anyone else when you don't nurture yourself. A burned-out, cranky husk of a woman can't be of much help to anyone. You can't give and give without ever replenishing. The key is to find a way to take better care of yourself first. Be the best that you can be for yourself and for your loved ones. For many of us, this represents a difficult shift in our core beliefs.

As women, we need to embrace the notion that our needs are at least as important as the needs of people we love. We have a responsibility to make ourselves a top priority. If we don't value ourselves and our own health, no one else will.

The Seven Keys ●●●

When you've invested so much of your time in caring for others, it's sometimes difficult to know where to begin taking care of yourself. Instinctively, many of us gravitate toward vegging out in front of the TV with a pint of ice cream or a bag of chips, but, truly, this is the exact opposite of self-nurturing. Ingesting large amounts of junk foods that will make our bodies feel (and, ultimately, look) worse is, in the end, a form of self-loathing and punishment.

We must make special time for ourselves every day with simple changes that will enhance the way we look and feel. There are seven keys to being fit and female. I use the acronym FEMALES to help my clients focus on these seven principles daily.

F: Find Something That's Fun

I'm astounded by the number of women who tell me they know that running (or spinning or aerobics or whatever) is good for them, but they really hate doing it. Here's a tip: if you truly hate doing something, don't do it. It doesn't matter why you hate it. The very fact that you hate something is reason enough not to do it.

Working out should be a pleasurable activity that you look forward to. Exercising may be difficult at first, and on some days you will certainly be more enthusiastic about it than on others. Overall, though, your fitness time should be your sanctuary, your private time, your play time. That's why it's so important to pick something you like—better yet, something you *love*—as your primary activity. Fortunately, there are plenty of enjoyable choices out there for women of every shape and size. For example, your muscular conditioning could include everything from yoga to Pilates to weight training with machines. Aerobic choices run the gamut from walking to in-line skating, from tennis to square dancing. (More on this in chapters 6 and 7.)

Whatever activity you choose, just make sure that there is an element of pure fun to it. Listen to your mind and your body. If you find something dead boring or totally uncomfortable, avoid it like the plague. Even women can only be so masochistic, so if you really hate something, it's highly unlikely that you'll stick with it.

E: Exercise Daily

Daily?!! you might think. Is she suggesting that I exercise every single day? I'll be lucky if I can do something two or three times a week.

Yes, as crazy as it sounds, that is exactly what I'm suggesting.

Here's why. Life being what it is, invariably something will come up and derail your exercise plans. This means that if you plan on working out only two or three days per week, whenever you miss a session you are down to working out only once or twice a week. Unfortunately, this isn't enough exercise for most of us to reach our goals. Schedule exercise daily, and in reality, you'll probably end up working out three to five times per week—the recommended amount. So plan on working out daily because, realistically, it won't actually happen every day.

Another key to success? Try to schedule your workouts in the morning, if possible. Studies show that morning exercisers are as much as 50 percent more likely to stick with their programs. Why? Perhaps because there are fewer distractions first thing in the morning. In a typical day, a million little things can go awry—the meeting that runs longer than expected, the lunch that didn't settle quite right, the phone call that you just had to make. By working out in the morning, you set yourself up for success, finishing your routine before all those everyday distractions thwart your exercise plans.

M: Muscle Toning

Most women I know just want to be thinner—they don't particularly care about having muscles. I have never had a female client, regardless of her shape, who told me that she wanted to get big, bulky muscles. That's a good thing, too, because even if a woman did want to turn into the Incredible Hulk, it's highly unlikely that she could. Most women don't have enough of the male hormone testosterone to end up looking like a side of beef. To get in the best shape of your life (and stay there), however, you will need to do some work enhancing your muscle tone.

After the age of thirty, women (and men) lose muscle mass at a rate of about 3 to 5 percent per year—and muscles make a very significant contribution to metabolism. In the previous chapter, I mentioned that every pound of muscle in your body burns about 30 to 50 extra calories per day. That may not sound like a lot, but the loss of even 1 pound of muscle tissue can result in a 5-pound body-fat gain in the course of a year. Not because muscles have turned into fat, but because the loss of muscle tissue has resulted in a steady weight gain from a decreased metabolism. In other words, you can continue to eat exactly what you always ate and experience a steady weight gain because you're burning fewer calories than you did before!

By increasing lean body tissue with resistance training, you not only prevent this frustrating scenario, you actually stoke your body's fat-burning furnace. And healthy muscles offer other benefits as well. They help maintain joint health, improve posture, prevent back pain, and add sexy curves to all the right places. From calisthenics to free weights, from machines to yoga, there are tons of enjoyable ways to improve muscle tone. The bottom line is that in order to be a lean, mean, calorie-burning machine, you'll need to commit to at least one body-sculpting activity and integrate it into your weekly routine at least twice a week.

A: Aerobics

Invariably, whenever I'm at a social gathering and people find out that I'm a personal trainer, someone in the room will ask how to get rid of "this." "This" is usually a handful of body fat on the person's waist or thighs. The individual always seems a little disappointed when I say that no exercise in the world will just burn fat from a certain body part. Sure, liposuction can remove fat from a particular place, but exercise doesn't work that way.

In other words, doing a million crunches won't burn fat off your middle, and doing a billion leg lifts won't reduce the size of your thighs. Unfortunately, we can't just sculpt the fat off the body parts we don't like. Fat has to come off the entire body, and that takes a commitment to regular cardiovascular exercise and a healthful diet. Although crunches and leg lifts will tone your muscles, if you don't reduce your overall body fat, those beautiful muscles will remain obscured by an extra layer of padding.

Some people call it aerobics, some call it cardiovascular exercise, and others call it "thirty minutes of hell on earth," but in one form or another, this kind of exercise needs to be a part of your weekly routine. While all body types require at least some cardiovascular exercise, if you are an endo-pear or an endo-apple body type, it's especially important to pick at least one type of cardiovascular exercise (but preferably a few) that you enjoy in order to sculpt your shape into the best that it can be.

L: Learned Selfishness

Years ago, before I was in the fitness business, I worked at various jobs in advertising and public relations. I remember a business associate of mine who was known for his habit of scheduling meetings around his workouts. Although I was exercising at the time, I can remember thinking how rude and selfish it was for this man not to make himself available during that specific time period. Even more outrageous, I thought, was the fact that he didn't even have the decency to tell a little white lie about it! He just matter-of-factly told anyone who asked that he wasn't available during his exercise time. Needless to say, this gentleman was always in great shape and vibrant good health.

Ironically, now that I'm a fitness professional, I don't consider this person selfish in the least. Today, I think of him as a genius—a role model. This man made a total commitment to his health and well-being in a way that few people ever do. His body and his health were top priorities. Best of all, he didn't feel the need to lie or apologize to anyone for it!

If you tell yourself that you'll exercise whenever you get a chance, I can pretty much guarantee that you won't exercise at all. There is always something that just pops up out of nowhere and monopolizes a woman's time: a phone call, an errand, something you need to do for the kids, a fascinating television program—whatever. If we don't take control and make our fitness time a priority and actually schedule our lives around it, exercise invariably ends up at the very bottom of the to-do list.

Again, morning is the ideal time for this, but if that's not workable, think of some part of your day when you can have a minimum of thirty minutes that is yours alone. Put any nagging guilt aside and remind yourself that you deserve to look and feel your best—not just for your own sake, but for all the people you care about. Put the world on hold for thirty minutes while you take care of yourself. You (and everyone else in your life) will be better off for it.

E: Eating Right Almost All the Time

If I tried to sell you a car that I told you wouldn't run 90 to 95 percent of the time, would you buy it? Of course, you wouldn't. Well, overall, diets have a 90 to 95 percent failure rate! Studies show that fewer than 5 percent of all dieters actually achieved their desired weight loss and kept it off for five years.

There are two major reasons for this. First of all, most diets don't teach people how to change their eating habits and maintain their weight loss in the long run. The focus is on the quick fix: lose a few pounds and then go back to eating as you did before.

Yet when you stop dieting, you return to the habits that resulted in the weight gain in the first place, and gradually the weight creeps back on.

The only way to break this cycle is to never "go on a diet" again. Instead, you must think about changing the way you eat each and every day! By following an eating plan that allows you to savor the pleasures of food while making more intelligent choices every day, you'll free yourself from the frustrating cycle of dieting. Knowing that it's a month before bathing suit season or two weeks before a friend's wedding will no longer be cause for panic.

S: Sleep as a Priority

We are one seriously sleepy nation. Experts find that most of us don't get the recommended seven to nine hours of sleep per night. Unfortunately, the health consequences of sleep deprivation are far more serious than just a few extra daytime yawns. Perpetual sleepiness leads to difficulty handling stress, slurred or fragmented speech, inability to control emotions, increased appetite that results in weight gain, deterioration of the immune system, compromised problem-solving ability, decreased muscle strength, and an increased tendency toward accidents, to name just a few things.

Worse yet, research on chronic sleep deprivation reveals that sleep-deprived people aren't fully aware of just how exhausted they are. They have become so used to running on too little sleep that they cannot tell how much their daily functioning is being compromised. In our 24/7 society, it's easy to develop what experts call a "sleep debt." Let's say, for example, that you get six hours of sleep per night, rather than the recommended eight; in the course of just two weeks, that will add up to twenty-eight missed hours of rest. That's the equivalent of three and a half nights of sleep! Not surprisingly, women tend to be even more behind in their sleep than the general population is.

The bottom line? There is no substitute for sleep. In order to function at your peak, with the level of health and vitality that you deserve, you are going to move sleep toward the top of your to-do list. Much like brushing your teeth and taking a multivitamin, adequate sleep needs to be considered an essential in your health-maintenance routine. Pick a reasonable bedtime that will get you seven to nine hours of healing sleep—and stick to it. Don't let Jay Leno or that extra load of laundry stop you from catching your zzzzs—your mind and body can't function properly without them!

It's Your Parents' Fault ●●●

Another key concept is genetics. For better or worse, you are what you are. If you want to know what you've inherited, take a look at your parents and siblings. Certain physical characteristics run in families. From eye color to hair texture, from height to ideal body weight, chances are you can look at Mom, Dad, Grandma, and Grandpa and figure out where your body parts came from.

For better or worse, these traits represent the hereditary hand that fate has dealt you. That's why it's wise to learn to love the genetic cards that you've been dealt. It is what it is. Embrace it, because you can't change it. Biology is destiny.

Let's say, for example, that you have short legs and tend to be a bit overweight. You can dramatically improve your appearance (and health) with a sound diet and exercise program, but you cannot develop longer legs.

Despite the advertised claims of many exercise programs, you cannot become longer from diet or exercise. Leaner, yes. Longer, no. Limb length has to do with the length of the long bones in your body, primarily the humerus and the femur. If you are a full-grown adult, you will not become longer from exercise. Exercise strengthens muscles, tendons, and bones. Exercise increases flexibility and range of motion. Exercise improves posture. But unless your first name happens to be Gumby, exercise won't change the length of your bones. If you have short femurs, you have short legs. If you have long femurs, you have long legs. Weight loss, diet, and exercise won't change the basics of what Mother Nature has given you. At your most fit, you will be a gorgeous, flawlessly conditioned specimen of a woman—with short legs. And guess what? That's okay.

How boring would it be if all women on the planet looked exactly the same? The natural differences in our body shapes give each of us our own special brand of beauty. Remember, you will always be disappointed with your body if you compare yourself to a woman who has a totally different inherited body structure. Try to tune out the stereotyped concept of feminine beauty and learn to embrace the physical attributes that make you *you*. A customized program of appropriate exercise and proper nutrition will give you powerful tools to sculpt your particular genetic gifts into your body's own version of perfection. Just be sure to measure your progress by your own yardstick. In the next chapter, we'll explore the six basic shapes that the female form comes in: the six female body types.

the six female body types: what shapes we come in

Sheldon's Somatypes ●●●

In the 1940s, an American psychologist named William Sheldon developed an interesting (if somewhat bizarre) method of classifying body types. He called his work "the Somatype Theory."

After studying photographs of thousands of men and women from all walks of life, Sheldon concluded that most human beings could be grouped into one of three categories: ectomorphs, mesomorphs, or endomorphs.

Unfortunately, Sheldon's theory didn't stop there. He also believed that by identifying a person's body type, you could predict his or her major personality traits. According to Sheldon, each of the three body types is controlled by a different physiological system, which dictates a particular psychological disposition.

Specifically, Sheldon held that (1) ectomorphs (dominated by the nervous system) are cerebral and introverted by nature, (2) mesomorphs (controlled by the musculoskeletal system) are physical and outgoing, and (3) endomorphs (under the influence of the digestive system) are relaxed and easygoing.

As you might imagine, this far-fetched aspect of Sheldon's work was soundly rejected by the scientific community. His descriptions of the three body types, however, have proven valid and useful and are still widely used today by health and fitness professionals alike. Here is a look at Sheldon's three somatypes in greater detail.

The Ectomorph

According to Sheldon, the ectomorph is small-boned, slender, and delicate, with narrow hips and shoulders. Ectomorphs are naturally thin, with high metabolisms, and have a problem gaining weight. Usually long-limbed, they tend to have small muscles and difficulty increasing muscle mass. Celebrity examples of this type would include Kate Moss, Gwyneth Paltrow, and Angelina Jolie.

The Mesomorph

The medium-framed mesomorph typically has a strong and fit appearance even if she doesn't exercise regularly. Mesomorphs are blessed with moderate to high metabolisms and seldom experience significant weight gain. They are natural athletes and develop impressive muscle tone without a lot of effort. High-profile examples of this type include Britney Spears, Angela Bassett, and Madonna.

The Endomorph

Larger-boned, and full-bodied, endomorphs tend to be round and shapely, even at their most fit. Endomorphs have slower metabolisms that cause them to gain weight easily and lose weight slowly. Fortunately, endomorphs can also gain significant muscle tissue with proper training. Of the three types, endomorphs vary the most in body size, ranging from being normal weight to being very overweight. Examples of endomorphs in the public eye run the gamut from Kate Winslet and Beyoncé Knowles to Carnie Wilson, Oprah Winfrey, Camryn Manheim, and Roseanne Barr.

Apples or Pears? ●●●

About the same time that Sheldon identified his somatypes, a French physician named Jean Vague began using his own system to classify body types. Vague believed that most people could be classified as either apples or pears. *Android* (or male-patterned) obesity was Vague's term for apple-shaped individuals who tend to hold extra weight in their midsections. *Gynoid* (or female-pattern) obesity was Vague's description for pear-shaped people, who gain weight in the lower body.

Vague's work was particularly significant because he was one of the first health professionals to observe that overall, "apples" experience greater health problems than "pears" do. Sixty years later, the medical community continues to investigate the role of apple-shaped obesity patterns in chronic disease processes, such as diabetes, coronary artery disease, cancer, hypertension, and stroke.

The Six Female Body Types

While the overwhelming majority of men are apples (with either endomorph, ectomorph, or mesomorph tendencies), there is a great deal more variation among women. Women can be apples or pears. Within those broad categories, women can also be ectomorphs, mesomorphs, or endomorphs.

That is why it's useful to use both Sheldon's and Vague's systems together to identify six major female body types: the endo-pear, the endo-apple, the meso-pear, the meso-apple, the ecto-pear, and the ecto-apple. Each body type has its own unique challenges—and its own advantages. Moreover, each body type requires a customized workout program and eating plan to maximize its potential. Let's look at each of the six body types in greater detail.

The Three Pear Types

From Marilyn Monroe to J-Lo, the pin-up girls of every generation have traditionally been pears. The reason is simple. Men love curves—and pears have them! Pears tend to have smaller waists, rounder bottoms, and fuller hips and thighs. Naturally shapely, pears often bemoan their curves, longing for the straight-up-and-down look of a fashion model.

To avoid being frustrated by their body type, pears need to understand that in general, there is a strong hormonal predisposition for women to deposit body fat in the lower body. For thousands of years, the survival of the human species has relied on the ability of women's bodies to store enough body fat in order to reproduce. The hips, the thighs, and the buttocks are gender-appropriate storage sites for the body fat needed for normal reproductive functions. In fact, the changes that occur during menopause can actually cause lifelong pears to turn into apples due to a loss of these female hormones.

The plus side of being a pear is that even at their heaviest, pears are less likely to have obesity-related health problems than apples are. On the downside, there is increasing evidence that body fat stored in the lower regions doesn't break down as easily as abdominal body fat does. This can frustrate pears in their efforts to trim down.

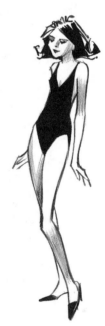

The Ecto-Pear

The typical ecto-pear is blessed with a warp-speed metabolism and rarely (if ever) gains weight. Naturally slender, with a hint of curves in the lower body, the ecto-pear has a difficult time increasing muscle mass, particularly in the upper body.

The training routine for the ecto-pear will focus on providing (1) enough cardiovascular exercise for heart health without promoting additional weight loss; and (2) higher-resistance, lower-repetition exercises for both upper and lower body to balance the proportions with lean muscle mass.

The Meso-Pear

This body type has a strong but feminine lower body, a well-defined waist, and a lean, slight upper body. Meso-pears tend to put on lower body muscle easily and often describe a tendency to bulk up from weight training. Typically of normal weight, meso-pears are seldom overweight or stick thin. To one extent or another, however, meso-pears will always have a bit of fullness through the hips, the thighs, and the buttocks. The healthy meso-pear will look fit and toned but never skinny. Therefore, it's important for meso-pears to embrace their tendency toward an athletic look with feminine lower-body curves.

The meso-pear training plan will focus on providing (1) sufficient low- to multi-impact cardio-vascular exercise, keeping body fat down; (2) lower-weight, higher-repetition resistance training for the lower body, to sculpt without bulk; and (3) higher-weight, lower-repetition resistance training for the upper body, to balance proportions with increased upper-body musculature.

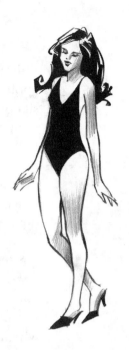

The Endo-Pear

Naturally curvaceous, the endo-pear tends to gain weight easily in the lower body. A particular challenge for the endo-pear is that even if she's super-fit, she will never look waiflike or chiseled. Moreover, because the endo-pear shape is not our culture's standard of perfection, examples of this body type are dramatically underrepresented in the media. That's why it's important for endo-pears to compare themselves to body-appropriate, real-world inspirations of endo-pear fitness and beauty. If they continually measure themselves against women with body types radically different from their own, unrealistic expectations, frustration, low self-esteem and even body-image disorders can result.

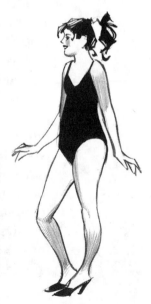

The endo-pear training program will focus on providing (1) plenty of low-impact cardiovascular training to keep body fat down; (2) lower-weight, higher-repetition resistance training to sculpt and define the lower body; and (3) moderate- to high-weight, lower-repetition resistance training to balance overall proportions with upper-body muscle tone.

The Three Apple Types

Although pin-up girls are usually pears, supermodels are almost always apples. Ever since Twiggy's domination of the runway in the 1960s, the slenderest apple body types have been the first choice of fashion designers.

Why? Because apples are blessed with long, lean legs, which photograph beautifully and show off fashions to their best advantage. In fact, even at their heaviest, apples still tend to have gorgeous gams. On the downside, many apples are frustrated by their attempts to chisel well-defined waistlines.

Of much greater concern is the fact that overweight apples are at greater risk for obesity-related health problems. These include adult-onset diabetes, cardiovascular disease, high blood pressure, and stroke. The good news for apples is that studies show that fat stored in the mid-section is more readily broken down with proper diet and exercise, which can make losing weight less difficult for apples than for their pear counterparts.

The Ecto-Apple

Like her ecto-pear sisters, the typical ecto-apple is blessed with a speedy metabolism. Naturally slender, with hardly any curves at all, the ecto-apple has the leanest appearance of all the body types. While ecto-apples rarely have a weight problem, they do have a difficult time increasing muscle mass and often perceive themselves as being scrawny or gawky. Because they are frequently undermuscled, maintaining good posture can be a particular challenge for this body type.

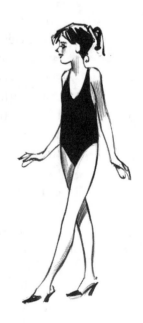

A training routine for the ecto-apple will focus on providing (1) enough aerobic exercise to promote heart health; and (2) moderate- to high-weight, low-repetition resistance exercises for the entire body, to build shapely muscles and improve posture.

The Meso-Apple

Meso-apples have sinewy, lean legs with natural softness through the midsection. This body type almost never gains weight (or bulk) in the lower body. However, even at their most slender, meso-apples have a hard time developing muscular definition in their abdominals. Thankfully, proper diet and physical conditioning can make this body type a true athletic inspiration.

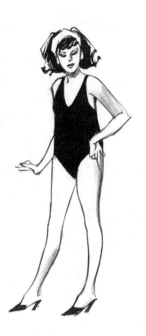

The training plan for the meso-apple will focus on providing (1) enough moderate low-impact (or multi-impact) cardiovascular exercise to help reduce body fat in the midsection; (2) higher-weight, lower-repetition resistance training for the lower body to help balance her proportions; and (3) low-weight, high-repetition resistance training for the upper body and the torso, to sculpt without bulk.

The Endo-Apple

The endo-apple tends to be full through the waist, the bust, and sometimes the upper arms but often with well-defined legs and a small, flat backside. It's very easy for this body type to gain weight through the midsection. Even at her appropriate thinnest, an endo-apple will never have a wasp waist. However, a sensible program of diet and exercise can radically alter endo-apple proportions and make her already "to die for" legs that much more impressive.

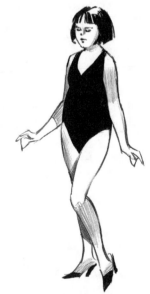

The endo-apple training program will focus on providing (1) lots of low-impact cardiovascular training to reduce overall body fat; (2) lower-weight, higher-repetition resistance training for the upper body and the torso to the midsection to increase definition; and (3) moderate- to high-weight, lower-repetition resistance exercise for the lower body to increase lower-body muscle mass and to balance proportions.

Defining Your Shape ●●●

After reading the previous descriptions, you'll probably have a good idea which shape best describes you. Are you still unsure? That's okay. Many women (including me) are actually a combination of two of the body types. There is, however, usually one body type that predominates.

If you still need a bit more convincing, the following chapter should remove any doubt, as you go through a step-by-step process to determine which body type is your perfect fit.

5

which woman are you?
finding your body type

E ach of my Fit + Female workouts in chapter 7 is specifically
designed to best meet the needs of a particular body type. Therefore, in order to get optimal results, it's important to determine which
body type best describes you.

This chapter will allow you to pinpoint your Fit + Female body type,
and it provides a quick and easy way of determining your current level
of fitness.

As you read through each item, select the answer that best describes
you. Keep in mind that there are no right or wrong answers. In order to
get the most out of your program, it's important to be as open and honest as possible. If you are unsure about a particular question or really
don't see an appropriate answer to a particular question, simply leave
that item blank.

Fit + Female Body Type Questionnaire

1. I tend to gain weight
   a) very easily/easily
   b) somewhat easily
   c) hardly ever
   d) never

2. I tend to get bulky if I weight train.
   a) True
   b) False

3. People would probably describe me as
   a) very thin/thin
   b) normal weight
   c) slightly overweight
   d) overweight

4. I have
   a) very little or no cellulite
   b) some cellulite on my hips, butt, or thighs
   c) a lot of cellulite on my hips, butt, or thighs
   d) some cellulite on my stomach

5. I have
   a) an hourglass figure
   b) a small waist and strong legs
   c) a small upper body and slender legs with a round butt
   d) a full bosom and very slender legs
   e) a straight-up-and-down waist and strong legs
   f) a slender body everywhere but a little bit of a belly

6. Compared to most other women, I would say my legs are
   a) thin or thinner than most
   b) average sized
   c) the largest part of my body

7. My breasts are
   a) C–D cup or more
   b) A–B cup

8. My butt is pretty flat; I wish it were rounder.
    a) True
    b) False

9. I tend to get varicose and/or spider veins in my legs.
    M **a)** True
    b) False

10. I have a long torso.
    a) True
    M**b)** False

11. No matter what I do, I always seem to have a bit of a belly.
    M **a)** True
    b) False

12. No matter what I do, I always seem to have a full butt and/or thighs.
    a) True
    M **b)** False

13. Throughout my life, people have always told me that I have great legs.
    M **a)** True
    b) False

14. Throughout my life, people have always envied my flat stomach and/or small waist.
    a) True
    M **b)** False

15. When I gain weight, I tend to gain it
    M **a)** in my waist
    b) in my hips

16. No matter what I eat, I never seem to gain weight.
    a) True
    M **b)** False

17. Most of the women in my family are somewhat bottom heavy.
    a) True
    M **b)** False

18. Most of the women in my family are very busty with skinny legs.
    a) True
    b) False

19. My doctor has told me that I am at risk for developing type 2 diabetes.
    a) True
    M **b)** False

20. Using a tape measure, measure the narrowest part of your waist and the widest part of your hips. Then divide the waist measurement by the hip measurement.
    a) The number was .80 or greater.
    b) The number was less than .80.

21. I typically work out at least three times per week.
    M **a)** True
    b) False

22. I do at least twenty minutes of cardiovascular exercise three to five times per week.
    M **a)** True
    b) False

23. I lift weights, use resistance-training equipment, or take a body-sculpting class two to three times per week.
    a) True
    M **b)** False

24. In the past year, I have
    M **a)** not gained any weight
    b) lost weight
    c) gained ten pounds or more

25. I can walk briskly, jog, dance, or ride a bike continuously for at least thirty minutes without becoming winded.
    M **a)** True
    b) False

26. After sitting quietly for at least ten minutes, use your index and third fingers to take a pulse on the thumb side of your wrist for one full minute. What was the number of beats in that minute?
    a) 70 or higher
    b) Between 70 and 60
    c) Below 60

27. I can bend down and touch my toes
    a) very easily
    b) somewhat easily
    c) with some difficulty
    d) not at all

28. I can do at least twenty full sit-ups in one minute (with my feet held down).
    a) True
    b) False
    c) Not sure

29. I could lift at least my body weight one time on the leg-press machine in the gym.
    a) True
    b) False
    c) Not sure

30. I could chest press at least half of my body weight one time on the chest-press machine in the gym.
    a) True
    b) False
    c) Not sure

31. I could do at least thirteen push-ups on my knees if I had to.
    a) True
    b) False

32. I could *definitely* jog (or brisk walk) one mile in less than seventeen minutes.
    a) True
    b) False

Answer Key

Now that you have completed the test, find the number or letter that corresponds to your answer for each item.

(handwritten margin notes: "Me-ec to pear", "Non-A meso-apple B.")

1. a) 4
   b) 3
   c) 2
   d) 1
   d) 4
   e) 3
   f) 1

2. a) 3
   b) 0

3. a) 1
   b) 3
   c) 4
   d) 4

4. a) 1
   b) 2
   c) 4
   d) 2

5. a) 4
   b) 3
   c) 1

6. a) A
   b) No score
   c) B

7. a) A
   b) B

8. a) A
   b) B

9. a) B
   b) A

10. a) B
    b) A

11. a) A
    b) B

12. a) B
    b) A

13. a) A
    b) B

14. a) B
    b) A

15. a) A
    b) B

16. a) A
    b) B

17. a) B
    b) A

18. a) A
    b) B

19. a) A
    b) B

20. a) A
    b) B

21. a) A
    b) B

22. a) T
    b) U

23. a) T
    b) U

24. a) T
    b) T
    c) U

25. a) T
    b) U

26. a) U
    b) T
    c) T

27. a) T
    b) T
    c) U
    d) U

28. a) T
    b) U
    c) U

29. a) T
    b) U
    c) U

30. a) T
    b) U
    c) U

31. a) T
    b) U

32. a) T
    b) U

Scoring

Now look at your answers and see which numbers and letters appear most frequently. Items 1 to 5 should allow you to determine whether you are endo, ecto, or meso; items 6 to 21 should allow you to determine whether you are an apple or a pear; and items 22 to 32 will determine whether you are a beginner or an advanced exerciser.

Test items 1–5

Mostly 4s and 3s: endo
Mostly 3s and 2s: meso
Mostly 1s: ecto

Test items 6–21

(handwritten: 6 A'S 6 B's)

Mostly As: apple
Mostly Bs: pear

Test items 22–32

Mostly Ts: advanced
Mostly Us: beginner

which exercises to do— and why

I always remind my clients that fitness is not "one size fits all." In order for any program to be effective, it needs to address the particular concerns of each individual woman's body type. Fitness professionals call this customization of a workout to suit each person the program design or the exercise prescription.

Although these terms may sound scientific, in actual practice this process is equal parts science and art. The science part of the equation involves understanding what each aspect does for the body. The art is tailoring each aspect to suit the specific needs of the individual.

In addition, while every program needs to be different, there are three key elements that must be included in any successful fitness program. Specifically, every woman (regardless of her body type) should have a regimen with these key elements:

A cardiovascular exercise component

A muscular fitness component

A flexibility component

Whenever a fitness program is unsuccessful, it's almost inevitably because one (or more) of the key elements wasn't there or too much effort was placed on one element at the expense of another.

Putting it another way, every successful program requires that all of the right "ingredients" are in the "recipe" and that they are added in the correct amounts.

Let's look at each of these key elements in closer detail, beginning with cardiovascular exercise.

Cardiovascular Exercise ●●●

When it comes to cardiovascular exercise, there are usually two types of women. There are those who love doing cardio (almost to the point of obsession), and those who would rather walk barefoot over a bed of hot coals than spend twenty minutes on a treadmill. Like it or not, though, regardless of body type, all women need at least some cardiovascular exercise to attain and maintain optimal health and wellness.

I am often asked whether something "counts" as cardiovascular exercise. By definition, in order to be cardiovascular exercise, the workout needs to

Be rhythmic in nature

Use the larger muscle groups of the body (principally the legs)

Elevate the heart rate into the target heart rate zone

Be performed over a sustained period of time (fifteen minutes or more)

Good forms of cardiovascular exercise include walking, bicycling, jogging, swimming, rollerblading, elliptical machines, stair machines, dancing, cross-country skiing, step aerobics, low-impact aerobics, and kickboxing classes.

Cardiovascular exercise has two primary benefits: strengthening the functioning of the heart, the lungs, and the blood vessels, and burning calories to promote weight loss and prevent weight gain.

For better or worse, most of my young, healthy female clients are not interested in how cardiovascular exercise will improve their health. Younger women are more concerned with how cardiovascular exercise will help them lose weight. It always reminds me of that old Billy Crystal routine from *Saturday Night Live* where he says, "I'd rather *looooook* maaaaarvelous, than *feel* maaaaaaarvelous." For most of these women, exercise (in general and cardio in particular) is merely a means to an end—a way of helping them look their best. And you know what? That's fine by me.

I'm happy to trick my clients into doing cardio for the aesthetic benefits, in the hopes that they will develop a healthy addiction to it—an addiction that could ultimately protect them from heart disease in the future. Because, although these twenty-, thirty-, and forty-something women may not care about this today, at some point in time they will.

Heart disease is the leading killer of women in the United States. Studies suggest that one in ten women between the ages of forty-five and sixty-four have some form of heart disease. After age sixty-five, that number jumps to one in four. One in twenty-five women will die of breast cancer, but one in two will die of a heart attack or a stroke. In other words, if you don't take good care of your heart when you're younger, you may not live to regret it.

Regular cardiovascular exercise protects against heart disease in many ways. The heart of a fit woman turns into a stronger, more efficient pump. Aerobic exercise increases the strength of the heart muscle overall, especially the left ventricle. The left ventricle is the most important chamber of the heart, because it's the one that's responsible for pushing oxygenated blood out into the rest of the body. A fit woman's heart fills more completely and pushes out more blood. This means that when a woman is cardiovascularly conditioned, her heart doesn't have to beat as rapidly or work as hard as it did before to do the same job.

Cardiovascular exercise helps to reduce blood pressure as well. In fact, the systolic (or the top blood pressure number) *and* the diastolic (the bottom blood pressure number) usually drop about 10 mmHg as a result of cardiovascular training. Having lower blood pressure means the heart doesn't have to strain against as much force in the arteries to push blood throughout the body.

Cardiovascular training also causes changes in the central nervous system. Aerobic activity actually enhances the body's natural ability to calm itself down, by increasing the activity of the parasympathetic nervous system. This is the same system that is activated when people use stress-reduction techniques, such as meditation and yoga. More activity from the parasympathetic system means lower heart rates and reduced stress levels, both of which are very heart-healthy.

Some other benefits associated with cardiovascular training include

Better utilization of oxygen by working muscles

Improved blood flow

Better lung function

Increased energy levels

Enhanced fat burning

Higher levels of good cholesterol (HDL)

Stronger bones, ligaments, tendons, and cartilage

And, of course, the primary reason that most women love cardiovascular exercise is that it makes it easier for them to lose weight (and keep it off) by burning extra calories.

Most cardiovascular activities burn between 6 and 10 calories per minute. The average cardio workout burns somewhere between 300 and 600 calories per hour, depending on which activity is performed and the intensity of the exercise. Best of all, the calorie-burning benefits continue even after the workout is over.

Following a workout, you continue to burn a greater number of calories at rest than you did before you worked out. This is known as excessive post oxygen consumption (EPOC) or exercise after-burn. After-burn can last anywhere from fifteen minutes to forty-eight hours after a workout and depends mostly on the intensity of the exercise. The more intense the workout, the longer the effects of the after-burn.

Common Cardiovascular Myths

There are a good many myths and misconceptions about cardiovascular exercise. What it is—and what it is not. What it can do for you—and what it can't. Test your own cardio-savvy as we examine each premise in detail.

"If you want to burn fat and lose weight, don't exercise too intensely. If you work out too hard, you'll burn mostly 'sugar,' not 'fat.'"

False (and true). This particular myth has gotten a lot of exposure from the heart rate charts that are typically displayed on various pieces of cardiovascular equipment.

Often, there will be a diagram printed right on a particular machine and the words *fat-burning zone* (or something like that) printed across the lower levels of intensity. In addition, there are usually a few workout programs within the machine with names like "fat burner" that use lower-intensity levels only. The reason this concept has gotten so much validation from the manufacturers of cardio equipment (and in magazines) is that it does have some basis in scientific fact.

It actually is true that the harder you exercise, the more sugar or carbs you'll burn during the actual workout. Overall weight loss however, is not dependent on what you burn while you exercise but rather is the result of the cumulative effects of negative energy balance.

In other words, if you burn more calories from a combination of exercise, an active lifestyle, and reducing your caloric intake, you will create a deficit. In order to make up for those extra calories that your body needs to function, your body will draw on its fat stores. So, even though more intense workouts do burn more sugar at the actual time of the exercise session, they burn more total calories as well. The greater the number of calories burned, the more the fat stores will be broken down and burned off to meet the body's energy needs.

In other words, all things being held constant, going at a higher intensity for a longer period will burn more total calories and will ultimately contribute to even greater weight loss. The key is, you can only work at those higher intensities if you are relatively fit. If you aren't as fit, you'll need to work at a lower intensity for a longer period of time.

"When working out to lose weight, remember that you have to work out for at least twenty minutes before you start burning fat."

True (and false). Technically, it is true that after twenty minutes, more calories are being burned from the breakdown of fats than from sugar. However, that's not the main reason to do cardio for longer than twenty minutes when you're trying to lose weight. The reason for this is simple: when you do more cardio, you burn more calories. Again, more calories burned overall is the goal when you're exercising to lose weight. Remember, the type of fuel that you're using at the time of the workout isn't the crucial factor—just try to burn as many calories as you can. Whether the calories come from fats or sugars, at the end of the day it doesn't matter. If you burn enough total calories overall, the extra that your body needs to function will be taken out of the fat stores.

"Three times per week for 20 to 30 minutes is plenty of cardio."

True (and false). The truth is that it depends on your body type and your goals. If weight loss is not a major issue for you (as is the case for the ecto-apple and the ecto-pear), then 20 minutes 3 times per week is enough to achieve the heart-healthy effects of cardiovascular exercise.

However, if you need to lose weight and/or have a harder time keeping it off (as is the case for the endo-apple and the endo-pear), or if you want to be in peak physical condition, then 20 to 30 minutes 3 times per week isn't going to cut it. For those goals, you'll need to do at least 30 minutes of cardio 3 to 5 days a week. (We'll get more into the specifics of this in chapter 7.)

"I must have had a great cardio workout because I was really sweating a lot."

False. First of all, excessive sweating (in and of itself) is not necessarily a good thing.

Second, sweating is not always an accurate indicator of whether you had a good cardiovascular workout. Excessive sweating may indicate a rigorous workout, or it can simply be a sign that you are exercising in too humid an environment.

The evaporation of sweat is the body's primary way of cooling itself. When humidity is high, the air is already saturated with water vapor. The more water in the air, the less water will evaporate off the skin's surface. When sweat clings to the body, the body temperature begins to rise dramatically. This can lead to potentially life-threatening conditions, such as heat exhaustion and heat stroke.

In fact, fit people do sweat more overall, and they start to sweat earlier in a workout than unfit people do. This adaptation is important because it enables the body to cool itself more efficiently.

Ideally, it's best to aid the body in the process of evaporation by dressing in layers. That way, as exercise intensity increases, you can peel off layers, exposing more skin to the air and helping the sweat evaporate and cool you.

"Don't use the —— machine—it will make your butt (or legs) bigger."

False. Cardiovascular exercise isn't resistance exercise. The primary goal of cardiovascular exercise is to elevate the heart rate and keep it elevated (within the target heart rate zone) for a prolonged period of time. This in turn strengthens the cardiovascular system and helps burn calories (which aids in weight control).

Certainly, there is some muscular toning associated with cardiovascular training, but cardio, by its very definition, consists of a high number of repetitions from the constant, consistent pumping action of the muscles. Performing exercises in sets with more than twelve repetitions is not associated with building muscle. When you perform cardiovascular exercise, you do many, many repetitions, far beyond anything that would cause an increase in muscle size. Furthermore, the amount of resistance (or tension) that your muscles work against when you do cardio is (or should be) very low.

Cardiovascular training is not associated with muscular hypertrophy, or bulking up. In fact, if you were trying to increase your muscle size, you would have to do just the opposite: use very heavy loads and do very few repetitions.

Weight gain and heavy resistance training, not cardio, cause an increase in circumference size. So try to ignore the latest bad press about a particular machine or the unsolicited locker room advice of the local gym blabbermouth. Just pick the workout (or, better yet, several workouts) that you most enjoy doing, and (as they say in the Nike ad) Just Do It!

"—— is the best possible cardio workout."

False. All other things being held constant, there is no one best cardio exercise for everyone. What makes any cardiovascular workout effective is that it (1) raises your heart rate above resting levels, and (2) keeps it elevated for an extended period of time to strengthen your cardiovascular endurance and burn calories. Beyond that, there are a myriad of machines and activities to choose from.

When choosing a cardiovascular exercise, ask yourself the following questions:

1. Is the cardio workout that you've chosen something that you have easy access to? For example, you probably shouldn't choose swimming as your primary form of exercise if the nearest pool is thirty minutes away. Pick an activity that's as convenient and easy as possible. Try to have at least one option that you can do easily at home. Then, regardless of the weather or last-minute changes in plans, you'll always have a way to work out. Some good at-home workout options include using a stationary bike, walking or jogging on a treadmill, working out with a DVD, or simply taking a brisk walk around the neighborhood.

2. Does anything hurt you when you do the exercise? Exercise shouldn't hurt—ever. Period. A temporary mild discomfort or a slight burning sensation in the muscle is fine and to be expected, but actual pain is something else entirely. Pain is the body's way of notifying you about damage to its structures. Don't ever ignore it.

   Always use common sense. If running, for example, makes your back and your knees ache, rather than wearing knee wraps, buying a back brace, and swallowing half a bottle of ibuprofen after the workout, choose another activity. It doesn't matter that running is supposedly what gave Cousin Roberta her perfect figure. Roberta is Roberta, and you are you. Respect your body, and make the choices that are right for you!

3. Most important, do you enjoy doing it? As I mentioned earlier, running (or the elliptical machine or whatever) could be the greatest cardiovascular exercise in the world, but if you hate it, the chances are you won't do it. It's human nature to avoid unpleasant experiences as much as possible. Instead, choose something that's enjoyable, something that you'll look forward to each day, not dread. That way, you'll set yourself up for consistency, and consistency is integral to getting results.

Even if you aren't crazy about the exercise at first, try to pick an activity that you think you could learn to enjoy. It always amazes me how many women who initially hated doing a particular cardiovascular exercise often learn to love it when they find the right exercise for them— and when they see and feel the results of regular cardiovascular training.

As long as it's not done to the point of injury or unhealthy obsession, I believe exercise should become a healthful addiction in every woman's life. The truth is that many women quite literally do become addicted to the pleasurable sensations they get from doing cardiovascular exercise because when you exercise rigorously, the body actually produces its own form of pain-killing opiate drugs called endorphins. These endogenous (or body-produced) drugs, which are similar in composition to morphine and heroine, are thought to be responsible for the so-called runner's high. And if you needed any more of a sales pitch for doing cardio, how's this? They are also associated with the pleasurable feelings one experiences after consuming chocolate or having sex. Can somebody point me to the elliptical machine?

Monitoring Intensity

When you do cardiovascular exercise, it's important to do it at a high enough intensity to provide a cardiovascular training effect. Work below that intensity and you may not get all the heart-healthy benefits that you could. Work above that intensity and (unless you are an elite-level athlete) you may not be able to sustain it.

There are several easy ways to know if you are working out either too hard or not hard enough.

The Talk Test

This is perhaps the easiest method to use, and it's surprisingly effective. While doing your cardiovascular exercise, you should be able to talk, but you shouldn't have enough breath to sing. If you're working out so vigorously that you can't speak, you're working too hard. Conversely, if you can belt out "The Star-Spangled Banner" with plenty of air to spare, you need to crank up the intensity.

The Rating of Perceived Exertion

You should feel that you are working out either "fairly light," "somewhat hard," or "hard." You should not feel that your efforts are either "very light" or "very hard." This middle area—feeling that you're working between fairly light and hard—represents the lower end and the higher end of the target zone for most people. Even more interesting is that if you add a zero to the number next to each rating it usually corresponds closely to your heart rate. For example, if you feel that you're working out fairly light, the number next to it would be 11. Add a zero to the end of that, and the number will be 110. Typically, that's close to the heart rate that most people have when they are working at this intensity.

How Hard Do You Feel This Exercise Is?

6		14	
7	very, very light	15	hard
8		16	
9	very light	17	very hard
10		18	
11	fairly light	19	very, very hard
12		20	
13	somewhat hard		

The Target Heart Rate Range

Heart rate is an excellent indicator of how hard you are working, although learning how to find and take your heart rate takes a bit of practice at first.

To calculate an appropriate heart rate training zone, it's a good idea to figure out what your true resting heart rate is. This means taking your heart rate for a full minute for three mornings the first thing after you wake up (assuming that you didn't wake with a start). Then take the average of those three mornings. This is your resting heart rate.

Resting heart rates usually vary between 60 and 100 beats per minute. Knowing where you fall in this range will allow you to calculate the most effective target range. Keep in mind that if you take any kind of medications that lower the heart rate, this isn't an appropriate method for you to use to monitor your intensity. People taking heart rate–lowering medications should consult with their doctors about the best way to figure out how hard they are working.

To take your heart rate:

1. With your palm up, place your first and second fingers only on the thumb side of your wrist. Press down gently with your fingers until you feel the pulse.

2. Start counting the number of beats in fifteen seconds. Begin with zero.

3. Multiply the number of beats by four. This will give you your heart rate for one minute.

Calculating Your Target Heart Rate Zone

1. Calculate your age-predicted maximal heart rate by subtracting your age from 220.

   For example: The age-predicted maximal heart rate for a thirty-five-year-old woman would be 220 – 35 = 185 beats per minute (bpm).

2. Calculate your heart rate reserve. This is the range between your maximal heart rate and your resting heart rate. This represents how many beats there are between the fastest and the slowest speeds that your heart beats. To figure out the heart rate reserve, subtract your resting heart rate from your maximal heart rate.

For example: If the thirty-five-year-old woman in the previous example had a resting heart rate of 70 beats per minute, to calculate her heart rate reserve you would subtract 70 from 185, or 185 – 70 = 115 beats per minute.

3. Calculate the top and the bottom numbers of your training zone. The intensity of your workout can range from very low, at 50 percent of your heart rate reserve, to very high, or 85 percent of your heart rate reserve. The more fit you are, the higher the intensity at which you can work out. People who are new to exercise should begin at an intensity that's usually between 50 and 70 percent of their heart rate reserve. Those who are already fit may work in the higher end of the percentages, usually between 65 percent and 85 percent of their heart rate reserve.

    Important Note: After you figure out the percentage of your heart rate reserve you must add your resting heart rate back in to figure out the high end and the low end of the training zone.

    For example: Let's say that our thirty-five-year-old woman is new to exercise, so we'll use the lower end of the training zone, between 50 percent and 70 percent. $115 \times .50 = 57.5$ and $115 \times .70 = 80.5$. Now we'll add her resting heart rate back in to both the top and the bottom number: $57.5 + 70 = 127.5$ bpm and $80.5 + 70 = 150.5$ bpm. This means that the woman's training zone would be between 128 and 151 bpm.

Muscular Fitness ●●●

To paraphrase the old adage, "Women do not live by cardiovascular training alone." Burning calories and improving the cardiovascular system are only part of the equation. As one of my clients was fond of saying, "Resistance training makes it hard, and cardio removes the lard." In other words, cardiovascular training helps to burn fat, but to tone the muscles underneath, you'll need to do at least some resistance training.

Muscular fitness training has gotten some bad press over the years from women who insist that it can (or at some point actually did) make them "big and bulky." Whenever my female clients tell me that they tried working out with weights or machines and got bigger or bulkier, I always say that (1) something other than weight training (such as not watching their diet or not doing enough cardio) was probably responsible for the increase in size, and/or (2) they were not training correctly for their body type. In other words, most likely they were emphasizing heavy weights and lower repetitions, when in fact they should have been focusing on lower weights and higher reps.

When done properly, resistance training for women usually does not cause any significant increase in muscle size. Even if you made a concerted effort to become big and bulky, it would be difficult. A growth in muscular size demands increased protein synthesis, which requires a good deal of testosterone, the male sex hormone. Women typically have one-tenth the amount of testosterone that men have, which means that they cannot realize the degree of increase in muscular size that men can.

Unfortunately, photos of women bodybuilders with extreme musculature have done a great deal to scare women away from lifting weights. What most people don't understand is that these women didn't end up looking this way by accident. They were actually trying very hard to achieve these results—and it's a full-time job.

Female bodybuilders work out every day with very heavy weights, using heavy loads and lots and lots of training volume (time spent at the gym) in an all-out effort to get a particular look that they want for competition. Moreover, some of these women take drugs, such as anabolic steroids, because even tons of training won't give them the increase in size that they want. Bottom line: the odds that an average woman, using a sensible, balanced program of resistance training, will end up looking like a side of beef are pretty much slim to none.

Also, for many years there was a cultural notion that any muscularity in women was undesirable or unattractive. Thankfully, over the last twenty years there has been a dramatic increase in the number of female media icons with great muscular definition. Women such as Linda Hamilton (in *Terminator II*), Madonna, Angela Bassett (in *What's Love Got to Do with It?*), Demi Moore (in *GI Jane* or *Charlie's Angels: Full Throttle*), and Hilary Swank (in *Million Dollar Baby*) have redefined the notion of sexy so that it now includes strong and sinewy. Women no longer have to fear that being "cut" or "defined" is synonymous with being unfeminine. Muscle tone is now considered a desirable part of feminine beauty. That's a very good thing, too, because muscular fitness training provides women with benefits that are far more than skin-deep. Specifically, muscular fitness training helps to

Promote bone strength and reduce the chances of developing osteoporosis

Strengthen joints and connective tissue

Develop functional strength for sports and the activities of daily life

Boost metabolism by increasing lean body tissue and decreasing body fat

Improve self-esteem and self-confidence

As is the case with cardiovascular workouts, there are a great many misconceptions about muscular fitness training. Follow along and test your resistance-training IQ.

"—— is the best way to tone your muscles."

False. Generally speaking, it's unwise to categorize any exercise as good or bad. Certainly, some exercises are better for some individuals than others are, and there is a correct way to perform every exercise. Ultimately, however, it's more a question of choosing the right exercise for a certain individual at a particular point in time.

It's usually a good idea to include a fair number of functional exercises in your muscular fitness program. Functional exercises are called that because they have a "transfer of training." In other words, it's important that your workout include plenty of exercises that prepare and condition you for the things you do in everyday life.

Functional training replicates real-world movements such as lifting a child out of a car seat, climbing stairs, or pulling something down off a shelf. Incidentally, these are usually the kind of movements that cause injuries if you're not conditioned and prepared for them. By preparing your body for the activities of daily living (also known as the ADLs), you not only receive the aesthetic benefit of looking great, you also prepare your body to be ready for whatever life throws at you.

"Doing lots and lots of repetitions of an exercise really tones you and helps burn fat off your trouble zones."

False. When it comes to the number of times you perform an exercise, it *is* possible to have too much of a good thing. Performing an exercise more than 20 times means that this resistance is too easy for you. In other words, if you can do an exercise 20 times (or more) without any strain, you aren't working against enough resistance to provide an "overload."

Overload means forcing the muscles to do more work than they are accustomed to. This will make your muscles stronger and more fit.

This is why body-sculpting classes are often ineffective. Lifting the same 3-pound dumbbells that you have been lifting in class for three years means that you are not improving. Your muscles are used to lifting those same 3 pounds. They don't have to make any further improvements in order to get the job done—and they won't.

"It's important to do lots of crunches in order to burn fat off your belly."

False. This is known as "the myth of spot reduction." Everyone wants to hear that we can target our exercise to burn fat off the body parts that we are unhappy with. Yet body fat comes off the body systemically, not just off the parts you'd like. This means that if you are an endo-apple, you could do crunches from now until doomsday and you'll be toning the muscles underneath the body fat but not burning off the fat on top.

Once again, it is cardiovascular exercise combined with diet—not crunches—that reduces the spare tire around your middle. Crunches are an excellent way to tone the abdominals underneath, but if your abs are obscured by an extra layer of body fat, no one will be able to see them.

"I've heard that doing —— exercise will build up your butt (thighs, etc.)."

False. There is no one exercise that will build up a specific body part. Rather, it is the amount of resistance (or weight) that you use to train with that could potentially increase muscle size. Then again, even under conditions where women are trying (using extreme measures) to increase size, their gains are much, much less than men's are.

In fact, in one research study, women and men were trying to increase both muscular strength and size. Interestingly, the results showed that the relative increases in strength were pretty much the same for both men and women. Men, however, experienced a 25 to 30 percent increase in muscular size during the twelve-week training period, while women had only a 2.5 percent increase in size—or about one-tenth as much as the men.

There are no bad exercises. Certainly, some are better for some individuals than others are, and some are more effective. However, there is no one exercise that with a moderate weight load is going to magically transform you into the Incredible Hulk. So don't even worry about it.

Flexibility Training ●●●

The last of the three essential keys is flexibility training. Flexibility training is a catch-all phrase for many different kinds of stretching. There are elements of flexibility training in many things, including yoga, Pilates, active isolated stretch, contract-release, proprioceptive neuromuscular facilitation (PNF), movement prep, and more.

Overall, though, flexibility can be divided into two basic categories: dynamic stretching and static stretching. Dynamic stretching is a type of stretching in which you gently and rhythmically move your joints through a full range of motion—in other words, a moving stretch—whereas with static stretching, you get into a position and hold the stretch without moving, allowing the muscles to relax and lengthen.

Both types of flexibility training are effective. However, it's my opinion that dynamic (or moving) stretches tend to be most effective in the beginning of a workout, because they prepare the muscles, the joints, and the central nervous system for the movements that you will do during the workout.

Static stretching, on the other hand, is great at the end of the workout because muscles are warmer and more supple. Static stretching releases muscular tension created during the workout. Postworkout flexibility training also allows you to stretch when the muscles are warm and pliable, which is the optimal time for stretching.

Keep in mind that everyone has his or her own natural degree of flexibility. If you aren't a human pretzel, you can probably blame your folks, because flexibility is largely determined by genetics. With a consistent stretching program, it's possible to make vast improvements in your flexibility and range of motion, but if you weren't born with a genetic predisposition to being hypermobile (very flexible), you won't ever be Gumby. And you know what? That's not a necessarily a bad thing.

Many women don't realize that when it comes to flexibility, it's possible to have too much of a good thing. Being too flexible can be just as dangerous as being inflexible. There is an ideal range of motion that should be possible at every joint in the body.

Ideally, you want each joint (and the muscles and the tendons that control it) to be able to move enough to adapt to sudden changes of position and the challenges of everyday life, but not so much that they are unstable. If a joint is too loose (as is the case in very flexible individuals), there is often not enough stability to protect it from an injury. So don't be too envious when you see another woman at the gym putting her body into seemingly impossible contortions, because being overly flexible puts you at increased risk of injury in the same way that being inflexible does.

A Word about Specificity ●●●

In fitness, there is a concept known as "specificity." Specificity simply means that the changes that you experience in a fitness program are the direct result of whatever your program focuses on developing. In other words, if you do something on a consistent basis, you will get good at it. It sounds obvious. It's a little bit like that old joke, "Who's buried in Grant's Tomb?" What do you think improves when you work at cardiovascular fitness? Answer: your cardiovascular fitness.

I'm amazed, though, at the number of people who do, say, yoga, for example (which develops flexibility and muscular fitness), and wonder why their aerobic capacity is not all that it could be. The answer is simply that they aren't doing an exercise modality that develops this capacity.

What's interesting about these three essential keys is that most people tend to focus on the very things that they are already good at. Flexible people gravitate toward yoga, people with a naturally high aerobic capacity focus on bike riding or jogging, and strong people get into weight training. Folks would be better served focusing on areas where they are weakest in order to develop the other components of physical fitness to their full potential.

Human nature being what it is, though, people find it more gratifying to do things they have a natural aptitude for, which is probably why most of us end up doing more of the things that we least need to do. If you are challenged by something, it's a pretty good indicator that this is an area in which you are weak, an area that could use more training and attention.

In the next chapter, we'll look at each body type, the ways that the three essential keys can be combined for each type, and the matched specific needs of each woman.

how to work out for your body type

L et's examine the workouts for the six body types in greater detail. For each one, I've provided guidelines for the cardiovascular exercise requirements and the specifics of the resistance workout. The flexibility component will be similar for all body types and is contingent more on one's level of flexibility than on one's shape.

Also, for each body type there are options based on your goals and time constraints. Each workout has several versions. The "bare-minimum workout" lets you know what is the minimum amount of effort you can put into your program and still expect to see results. The next level is the "ideal workout," which is the one that in a perfect world would ensure that you meet your goals as quickly as possible. Finally, there is the "gung-ho workout," for overachievers who like to go above and beyond what is required, for even greater gains.

All of the exercises listed for each body type are illustrated at the end of this chapter. I suggest that you photocopy your particular workout game plan so that you can reference it easily and make notes on the pages about any tips and strategies you may want to keep in mind. Now let's look at each Fit + Female workout in greater detail.

Carla, the Ecto-Pear ●●●

At six feet tall and 125 pounds, Carla is one seriously skinny chick. When Carla came to me she was very frustrated because people always asked her whether she had an eating disorder—she doesn't. Yet every day she endures rude stares and thoughtless comments, like, "Oh, my God, you're emaciated!" or "Don't you eat?!"

The fact is, Carla not only eats—she eats a lot! During our initial consultation, she told me it had always been impossible for her to put on weight. Her daily routine includes eating at least 3,000 calories and running three to five miles. When I asked her why she was running so much, she said that she was trying to increase her muscle mass. I explained to Carla that too much running can actually decrease muscle mass—and it burns a whopping 300 to 500 calories a day in the process! In other words, Carla's workouts were doing the exact opposite of what she wanted.

In order for Carla to build up her slender frame, she would need to focus on weight training with challenging loads and cut way back on her running. We also had to analyze her diet to be sure that she was getting plenty of nutrients and sufficient calories to keep pace with her warp-speed metabolism.

Training the Ecto-Pear Body Type

Ecto-pears are typically concerned with gaining weight or at least maintaining the body weight that they have and filling out their slender frames with shapely muscle tone.

Cardiovascular Fitness Guidelines for the Ecto-Pear

Ecto-pears need to be especially careful not to overdo aerobic (also known as cardiovascular) exercise. The reason is that aerobic workouts burn calories like crazy, and the ecto-pear's metabolism is already a calorie-burning powerhouse. The cardio component of the ecto-pear program will include just enough aerobic fitness to ensure optimal health and wellness, without facilitating additional weight loss.

The Fit + Female Cardio Rx for the Ecto-Pear

All three workout levels for the ecto-pear ("bare-minimum," "ideal," and "gung-ho") will have the same 20 minutes of cardiovascular exercise 3 times per week. The best choice of aerobic activities for the ecto-pear include walking, bicycling, swimming, and light jogging, all of which can easily be done at lower to moderate intensities.

It certainly is possible for the "cardio-crazed" ecto-pear to do more aerobics or higher intensities than this; however, she must be sure that she consumes enough extra calories each day to compensate for the increased energy expenditure of her more intense workouts. A good rule of thumb for the ecto-pear is to add at least 100 calories to her diet for every 10 minutes of rigorous exercise, to ensure that her cardio workouts don't undermine her efforts to fill out her frame.

Muscular Fitness Guidelines for the Ecto-Pear

Ecto-pears (like their ecto-apple sisters) don't have to be concerned with bulking up from weight training, even when they use challenging loads. Such routines are unbeatable for adding beautiful muscular development to their slim structures.

Therefore, the cornerstone of the ecto-pear training program focuses on weight workouts using heavier weight loads and fewer repetitions (6–12 repetitions per set). The muscular fitness workout for the ecto-pear features power moves that recruit the maximal amount of muscle tissue with every repetition.

The Fit + Female Muscular Fitness Rx for the Ecto-Pear

The Bare Minimum Workout: 1 set, 2 times per week (6–12 repetitions of each exercise per set). Approximately 20 minutes.

The Ideal Workout: 2 sets, 2–3 times per week (6–12 repetitions of each exercise per set). Approximately 30–40 minutes.

The Gung-Ho Workout: 3 sets, 3 times per week (6–12 repetitions of each exercise per set). Approximately 1 hour.

Exercises For The Ecto-Pear ●●●

SQUATS

(tones the buttocks, the front and the back of the thighs, and the calves)

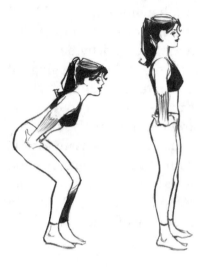

Stand with your feet hip-width apart, allowing for your natural turnout in the hips. Keeping the weight back on your heels, push your buttocks backward while reaching forward with your upper body. Your arms may be down or reaching out in front of you for balance. Bend until there is a 45- to 90-degree angle in your knees. Return to the starting position. Inhale on the way down and exhale on the way up.

SAFETY TIP: Make sure that you feel this exercise only in the thighs and the buttocks. If you feel strain in your knees, make sure that your weight is back on your heels and that your knees stay behind your toes at all times.

STEP-UPS

(tones the buttocks, the front and the back of the thighs, and the calves)

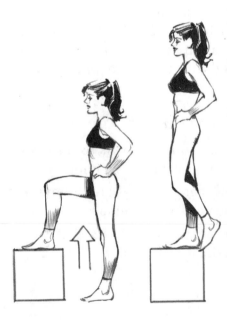

Stand with one foot on a sturdy bench or a step that's 6 to 12 inches high (the right step height for you should cause a 90-degree bend at your knee when you place your foot on it). Put all of your body weight on that same foot and, using your buttocks and thigh muscles, pull your body weight up on the step so that the other foot touches the step as well. Slowly lower yourself back to the starting position with a controlled movement. Exhale on the way up and inhale on the way down.

SAFETY TIP: Make sure that you feel this exercise only in the thighs and the buttocks. If you feel strain in your knees, make sure that your weight is back on your heels and that your knees stay behind your toes at all times.

PERFORMANCE TIP: Be sure not to use momentum to pull yourself up or lower yourself back down.

PUSH-UPS

(tones the chest, the shoulders, and the back of the upper arms)

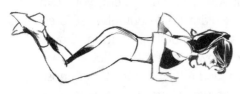

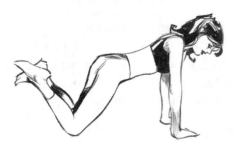

Kneel on a mat or a padded surface and place your hands on the floor about 6 to 8 inches away from your body, with your fingertips forward. Your hands should align with the nipple line of your chest. With a controlled motion, slowly bend your elbows and lower your chest toward the ground. Stop when each elbow is at a 90-degree bend. Then press back up to the starting position. Exhale as you push up and inhale as you lower yourself down.

SAFETY TIP: Don't lock your elbows out at the top or use momentum.

PERFORMANCE TIP: Keep your back flat, your abdominals tight, and your buttocks squeezed together. Keep the weight on the heels of your hands.

ROWS

(tones the back muscles and the front of the upper arms)

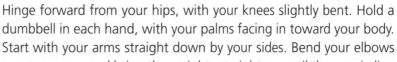

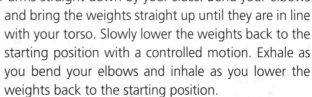

Hinge forward from your hips, with your knees slightly bent. Hold a dumbbell in each hand, with your palms facing in toward your body. Start with your arms straight down by your sides. Bend your elbows and bring the weights straight up until they are in line with your torso. Slowly lower the weights back to the starting position with a controlled motion. Exhale as you bend your elbows and inhale as you lower the weights back to the starting position.

SAFETY TIP: Protect your back by keeping your spine straight while at a 45-degree angle with the floor. Keep your abdominals drawn in tight and slightly bend your knees. If you cannot keep your back from rounding, place one hand on a chair back for support and perform the exercise one arm at a time.

PULLOVERS

(tones the chest, the back muscles, and the back of the upper arms)

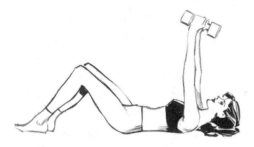

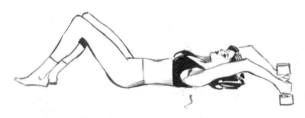

Lie on your back with your knees bent, your feet flat on the floor. Hold a single dumbbell securely with both hands over your belly button. Slowly lower the weight down toward the floor with a controlled motion, and return to the starting position. Inhale as you lower the weight over your head and exhale as you return it to the starting position.

SAFETY TIP: Keep your abdominals pulled in at all times and your lower back pressed down into the floor. Lower the weight slowly and with a controlled motion. Don't use momentum in either direction.

DIPS

(tones the back of the upper arms)

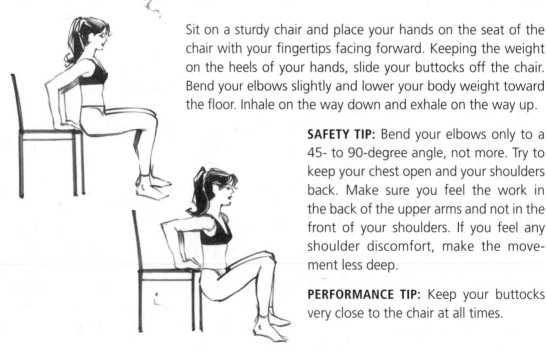

Sit on a sturdy chair and place your hands on the seat of the chair with your fingertips facing forward. Keeping the weight on the heels of your hands, slide your buttocks off the chair. Bend your elbows slightly and lower your body weight toward the floor. Inhale on the way down and exhale on the way up.

SAFETY TIP: Bend your elbows only to a 45- to 90-degree angle, not more. Try to keep your chest open and your shoulders back. Make sure you feel the work in the back of the upper arms and not in the front of your shoulders. If you feel any shoulder discomfort, make the movement less deep.

PERFORMANCE TIP: Keep your buttocks very close to the chair at all times.

BICEP CURLS

(tones the front of the upper arms)

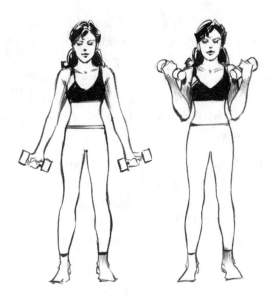

Stand straight and tall, holding a dumbbell in each hand. Your knees should be slightly bent, with your abdominals pulled in, your chest lifted, and your shoulders back. Bending only from the elbows, raise the weights up toward your shoulders. Keep your elbows in toward your side; don't use momentum in your arms. Don't move your back. Exhale as you raise the weights up and inhale as you lower them back down.

PERFORMANCE TIP: Be sure to lower the weights back to the starting position slowly and with a controlled motion.

REVERSE FLYS

(tones the middle of the back and the back of the shoulders)

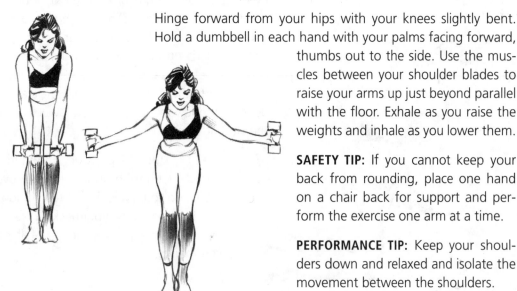

Hinge forward from your hips with your knees slightly bent. Hold a dumbbell in each hand with your palms facing forward, thumbs out to the side. Use the muscles between your shoulder blades to raise your arms up just beyond parallel with the floor. Exhale as you raise the weights and inhale as you lower them.

SAFETY TIP: If you cannot keep your back from rounding, place one hand on a chair back for support and perform the exercise one arm at a time.

PERFORMANCE TIP: Keep your shoulders down and relaxed and isolate the movement between the shoulders.

LOWER-BACK LIFTS

(tones the postural muscles that run along the spine)

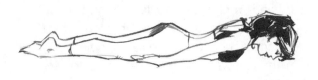

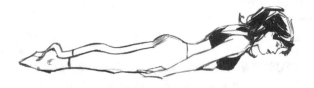

Lie facedown on a mat or a padded surface. Put your arms alongside your body, palms facing upward. Keep the area from your waist down pressed into the floor and lift from the waist up, just a few inches off the ground. Exhale as you lift and inhale as you lower.

SAFETY TIP: Be sure to look straight down at the floor to protect your neck. Don't come up too high; you should feel only the muscles alongside your spine working, without any pinching or discomfort at all.

ABDOMINAL CRUNCHES

(tones the abdominals)

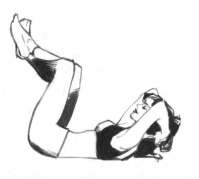

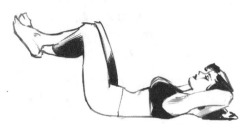

Lie on your back with your knees bent, your feet crossed at the ankles, and your hands placed gently behind your head. Lift your upper body and your legs up and in toward the center of your body at the same time. Then slowly lower them back to the starting position. Exhale as you bend your body and inhale as you lower back to the starting position.

SAFETY TIP: Keep your abdominals pulled in tight throughout the movement and your lower back pressed down into the floor. Keep your neck relaxed by letting the weight of your head fall into your hands.

Rebecca, the Meso-Pear ●●●

Rebecca is a natural athlete, strong and fit looking. She came to me for advice on how to make her powerful legs look slender and more in proportion to her small waist and upper body. "I feel like I'm all legs," she told me, "and whenever I exercise to make them look smaller, they seem to get even bigger than before!" It turned out that the mainstay of Rebecca's workout was lower-body weight training with machines, using heavy loads and few repetitions.

I explained to Rebecca that she was a meso-pear, with an exaggerated hourglass shape and a predisposition to gain both body fat and muscle easily in the lower body. To sculpt and define her legs, she would need to use light weights and higher repetitions. For her upper body, she would have to implement a program of heavier weights and fewer repetitions to increase muscle size and balance out her proportions. Finally, we needed to look at her cardiovascular exercise and diet to make sure that she was keeping her body fat at appropriate levels.

Training the Meso-Pear Body Type

This body type has a strong but feminine lower body, a well-defined waist, and a lean, slight upper body. Meso-pears put on lower body muscle easily and often describe a tendency to bulk up from weight training.

To one extent or another, meso-pears will always have a bit of fullness through the hips, the thighs, and the buttocks. Even if meso-pears are of normal weight (and they usually are), whatever storage body fat they have usually ends up below the waist. Before beginning any training program, meso-pears need to appreciate that even at their most fit they will never have skinny legs. Fit, toned, fabulously female, sexy as all get-out—but not skinny. This is the genetic hand that meso-pears have been dealt. And all things considered, it's not a bad one.

Mother Nature has designed all women to hold some extra body fat somewhere in order to ensure the survival of the species. Meso-pear (and endo-pear) body types hold that fat almost exclusively in the legs and the bottom. Although meso-pears may stare at images of Kate Moss and bemoan their fate, from a health perspective having a pear shape is actually a good thing. The reason is that as a group, meso-pears (and their endo- and ecto-pear sisters) are much less likely to suffer from many chronic diseases that are associated with having an apple physique. These maladies include heart disease, type 2 diabetes, stroke, and female cancers.

Also, meso-pears just naturally have more muscle tissue in their legs and thighs. That is not going to change. So, rather than curse their fate, meso-pears need to work on making their muscular legs strong and sinewy, toned but not overdeveloped.

Unfortunately, because an exaggerated pear shape is not the ideal image presented in the fashion pages, meso-pears (and endo-pears, for that matter) are often prone to body-image dissatisfaction—even eating disorders. To avoid unrealistic expectations and frustration, meso-pears must fully embrace their natural inclination toward a womanly, athletic look before starting on a fitness regime.

That said, with proper training the meso-pear can expect to (1) reduce the overall size of her lower body; (2) sculpt her hips, thighs, and buttocks; and (3) have better total body symmetry.

Cardiovascular Fitness Guidelines for the Meso-Pear

Meso-pears must also include a fair amount of cardiovascular exercise to help keep the body fat that's stored in the legs in check. Extra body fat is stored in the legs in two ways: under the skin (subcutaneously) and inside the muscle (intramuscularly), so it can make a significant contribution to the overall girth of the legs. If meso-pears reduce their body fat (within healthy levels), they will reduce the overall size of their lower bodies.

When choosing aerobic activities, meso-pears should select low-impact workouts because their larger hip size and greater lower-body mass can predispose them to injuries in the knees, the lower legs, and the feet. The best choices of aerobic activities for the meso-pear include power walking, bicycling, elliptical machines, stair climbing, and cardio kickboxing.

The Fit + Female Cardio Rx for the Meso-Pear

The Bare Minimum Workout: 20 minutes, 3 times per week

The Ideal Workout: 30–45 minutes, 3–5 times per week

The Gung-Ho Workout: 45–60 minutes, 3–5 times per week

Muscular Fitness Guidelines for the Meso-Pear

The training regimen for the meso-pear will focus on (1) lower-body resistance training with light weights and higher repetitions to tone the legs without bulk, and (2) upper-body resistance training with heavier weights and fewer repetitions to enhance upper-body proportions.

The Fit + Female Muscular Fitness Rx for the Meso-Pear

The Bare Minimum Workout: 1 set, 2 times per week (15–20 repetitions of the lower-body exercises [indicated with an *] and 6–12 repetitions of all other exercises). Approximately 25 minutes.

The Ideal Workout: 2 sets, 2–3 times per week (15–20 repetitions of exercises with an * and 6–12 repetitions of all other exercises). Approximately 30–40 minutes.

The Gung-Ho Workout: 3 sets, 3 times per week (15–20 repetitions of exercises with an * and 6–12 repetitions of all other exercises). Approximately 50 minutes to an hour.

SQUAT-SIDE LEG LIFTS*

(tones the buttocks, the front and the back of the thighs, and the outer thighs)

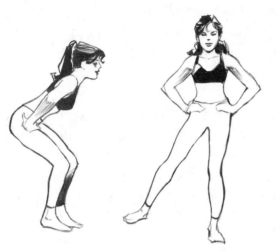

Stand with your feet hip-width apart, toes forward, allowing for your natural turnout in the hips. Bend your knees and push your buttocks backward, keeping the weight on your heels. As you return to the starting position, lift one leg out to the side, keeping the toes pointed forward. Raise the side of the leg toward the ceiling. Lower the leg back down and repeat, this time lifting the other leg. Exhale as you lift the leg and inhale as you lower.

PERFORMANCE TIP: Keep your torso upright and try not to lean over to the opposite side as much as possible.

PLIES*

(tones the buttocks, the front of the thighs, and the inner thighs)

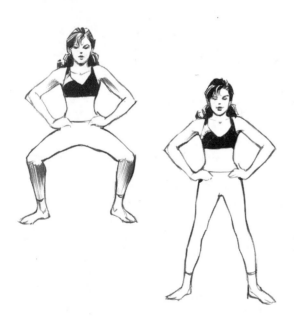

Stand with your legs turned out naturally from the hips. Your knees and toes should be in the same line. Bending at the knees and the hips, lower your buttocks straight down toward the floor until your knees are at a 45-degree angle. Slowly straighten your legs and return to the starting position. Exhale as you straighten your legs and inhale as you bend them.

SAFETY TIP: Make sure that you feel the work in the thighs and the buttocks and not in the knees. If you feel any discomfort in the knees, make sure that you aren't going down too far and that your knees and feet are in the same line.

LUNGE-BACKS*

(tones the front and the back of the thighs and the buttocks)

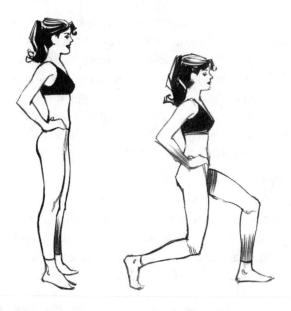

Start by standing tall with your feet hip-width apart. Step back with one leg and bend both your front and back legs so that the knees both make right angles. Using the muscles in the front leg, pull yourself up to the starting position. Inhale as you lower and exhale as you lift.

SAFETY TIP: Make sure that your front knee stays behind your front toes. Be sure that you feel the movement in the thighs and the buttocks and have no discomfort in the knees.

PUSH-UPS

(tones the chest, the shoulders, and the back of the upper arms)

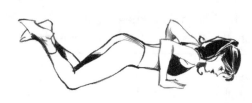

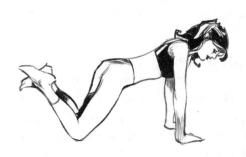

Kneel on a mat or a padded surface and place your hands on the floor about 6 to 8 inches away from your body, with your fingertips forward. Your hands should align with the nipple line of your chest. With a controlled motion, slowly bend your elbows and lower your chest toward the ground. Stop when each elbow is at a 90-degree bend and press back up to the starting position. Exhale as you push up and inhale as you lower yourself down.

SAFETY TIP: Don't lock your elbows out at the top or use momentum.

PERFORMANCE TIP: Keep your back flat, your abdominals tight, and your buttocks squeezed together. Keep the weight in the heels of your hands.

ROWS

(tones the back muscles and the front of the upper arms)

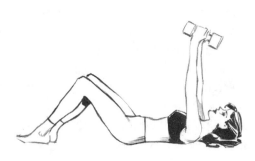

Hinge forward from your hips, with your knees slightly bent. Hold a dumbbell in each hand, with your palms facing in toward your body. Start with your arms straight down by your sides. Bend your elbows and bring the weights straight up until they are in line with your torso. Slowly lower the weights back to the starting position with a controlled motion. Exhale as you bend your elbows and inhale as you lower the weights back to the starting position.

SAFETY TIP: Protect your back by keeping your spine straight while at a 45-degree angle with the floor. Keep your abdominals drawn in tight and slightly bend your knees. If you cannot keep your back from rounding, place one hand on a chair back for support and perform the exercise one arm at a time.

PULLOVERS

(tones the chest, the back muscles, and the back of the upper arms)

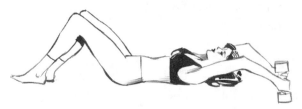

Lie on your back with your knees bent and your feet flat on the floor. Hold a single dumbbell securely with both hands over your belly button. Slowly lower the weight down toward the floor with a controlled motion, and return to the starting position. Inhale as you lower the weight over your head and exhale as you return to the starting position.

SAFETY TIP: Keep your abdominals pulled in at all times and your lower back pressed down into the floor. Lower the weight slowly and with a controlled motion. Don't use momentum in either direction.

DIPS

(tones the back of the upper arms)

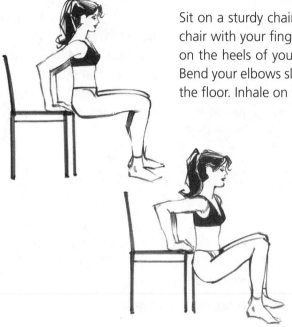

Sit on a sturdy chair and place your hands on the seat of the chair with your fingertips facing forward. Keeping the weight on the heels of your hands, slide your buttocks off the chair. Bend your elbows slightly and lower your body weight toward the floor. Inhale on the way down and exhale on the way up.

SAFETY TIP: Bend your elbows only to a 45- to 90-degree angle, not more. Try to keep your chest open and your shoulders back. Make sure you feel the work in the back of the upper arms and not in the front of your shoulders. If you feel any shoulder discomfort, make the movement less deep.

PERFORMANCE TIP: Keep your buttocks very close to the chair at all times.

BICEP CURLS

(tones the front of the upper arms)

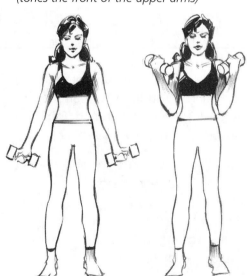

Stand straight and tall, holding a dumbbell in each hand. Your knees should be slightly bent, with your abdominals pulled in, your chest lifted, and your shoulders back. Bending only from the elbows, raise the weights up toward your shoulders. Keep your elbows in toward your side; don't use momentum in the arms. Don't move your back. Exhale as you raise the weights up and inhale as you lower them back down.

PERFORMANCE TIP: Be sure to lower the weights back to the starting position slowly and with a controlled motion.

REVERSE FLYS

(tones the middle of the back and the back of the shoulders)

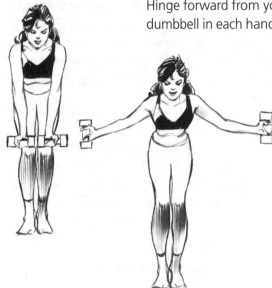

Hinge forward from your hips with your knees slightly bent. Hold a dumbbell in each hand with your palms facing forward, thumbs out to the side. Use the muscles between your shoulder blades to raise your arms up just beyond parallel with the floor. Exhale as you raise the weights and inhale as you lower them.

SAFETY TIP: If you cannot keep your back from rounding, place one hand on a chair back for support and perform the exercise one arm at a time.

PERFORMANCE TIP: Keep your shoulders down and relaxed and isolate the movement between the shoulders.

LOWER-BACK LIFTS

(tones the muscles that run along the spine)

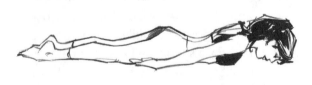

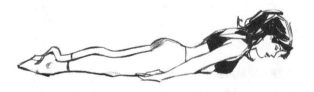

Lie facedown on a mat or a padded surface, with your arms alongside your body, palms facing upward. Keep the area from your waist down pressed into the floor and lift from the waist up, just a few inches off the ground. Exhale as you lift and inhale as you lower.

SAFETY TIP: Be sure to look straight down at the floor to protect your neck. Don't come up too high; you should feel only the muscles alongside your spine working, without any pinching or discomfort at all.

PELVIC BRIDGES*

(tones the buttocks, the back of the thighs, and the abdominals)

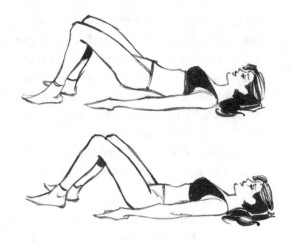

Lie on a mat or a padded surface on your back, with your knees bent and your feet flat on the floor. Keeping your head, neck, and shoulders down on the mat, lift your buttocks and the backs of your legs until your torso makes a 45-degree angle. Pause and squeeze at the top of the movement and slowly lower down to the starting position. Exhale as you lift and inhale as you lower.

FROG PRESSES*

(tones the inner thighs and the abdominals)

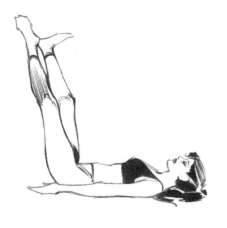

Lie on your back on a mat or a padded surface. Raise your legs up to 90 degrees, keeping your lower back pressed down. Rotate your thighs outward from the hips so that your heels touch each other and your toes point outward. Keeping the heels in constant contact with each other and the hips rotated out, draw the heels in toward your body as far as is comfortable and then push straight up. Inhale on the way in and exhale on the way up.

SAFETY TIP: If you feel any discomfort in your lower back, skip this exercise until your abdominal strength improves. Focus on pelvic bridges and bicycles instead.

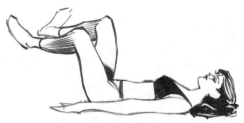

BICYCLES

(tones abdominals)

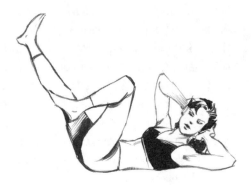

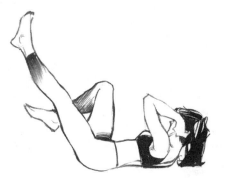

Lie on your back on a mat or a padded surface with your legs lifted at a 45-degree angle. Draw your right knee in toward your chest as you bring your left armpit toward your right knee. Then return to the starting position and draw your left knee toward your chest and your right armpit toward your knee. Alternate between these two positions, almost as if you were riding on a bicycle.

SAFETY TIP: Do only as many of these as you can without feeling any strain in your neck or lower back.

PERFORMANCE TIP: Be sure to keep your abdominals drawn in and your lower back pressed down into the floor.

Jessica, the Endo-Pear ●●●

Jessica has the body of a 1950s pin-up girl—voluptuous, with a true hourglass figure. At our first meeting, Jessica expressed some pretty unrealistic expectations about what her curvaceous frame should or could look like. She told me that she wanted to have a body "more like Gwyneth Paltrow's or Nicole Kidman's." As part of her ongoing quest, once or twice a year Jessica would get very motivated to "get in great shape." Her so-called health kick consisted of eating about 1,000 calories a day and working out for at least two hours every day. Typically, Jessica would stay on this program for a week or two, lose a few pounds, and then fall off the wagon. She wanted to know how to stay with the plan so that she could look the way she wanted to, once and for all.

I explained to Jessica that as an endo-pear, the last thing she should do is starve herself or overexercise. Not only was her fitness routine punishing and unhealthful, she was destroying lean body tissue, which would make her much more likely to gain weight in the future.

Over the next several months, we developed a balanced program of diet and exercise that Jessica could stay with (and actually enjoy) for the long haul. More important, we worked on getting Jessica some inspirational (yet realistic) endo-pear role models to look up to.

Training the Endo-Pear Body Type

Naturally curvaceous, the endo-pear is rounder on the bottom and smaller at the waist, with some fullness at the top. When endo-pears gain extra weight, it's concentrated in the hips, the thighs, and the buttocks.

A particular challenge for the endo-pear is to appreciate that even if she's super fit, she will never look waiflike or chiseled. Furthermore, because the endo-pear shape is not our culture's standard of perfection, examples of this body type are drastically underrepresented in the media. That's why endo-pears need to choose appropriate role models. Women such as Beyoncé Knowles, Catherine Zeta-Jones, or Jennifer Lopez illustrate that fit females needn't be skinny—or straight up and down. If endo-pears continually measure themselves against women who have shapes radically different from their own, the result can be unrealistic expectations, frustration, low self-esteem, and even body-image disorders.

Suitable endo-pear fitness goals include (1) toning and streamlining their womanly curves; (2) achieving and/or maintaining healthy, appropriate body fat levels; and (3) cultivating a healthy self-appreciation.

Cardiovascular Fitness Guidelines for the Endo-Pear

Because of her genetic predisposition toward weight gain, cardiovascular exercise is the cornerstone of the endo-pear's workout program. Aerobic workouts (in combination with muscular fitness and eating right) are unbeatable for keeping body fat at healthy and appropriate levels. It's important for the endo-pear to choose low-impact cardiovascular activities, particularly if she is overweight, because (1) they put less stress on the joints, and (2) they allow for longer/more frequent workouts with low risk of injury.

The best cardiovascular activities for endo-pears include power walking, stepping, low-impact aerobics, bicycling, spinning, and kickboxing.

The Fit + Female Cardio Rx for the Endo-Pear

The Bare Minimum Workout: 30 minutes, 3 times per week

The Ideal Workout: 45 minutes, 3–5 times per week

The Gung-Ho Workout: 45–60 minutes, 3–5 times per week

Muscular Fitness Guidelines for the Endo-Pear

The muscular fitness routine for the endo-pear will focus on lower-weight, higher-repetition resistance training (12–20 repetitions per set) to sculpt the entire body, with special emphasis on lower-body toning.

The Fit + Female Muscular Fitness Rx for the Endo-Pear

The Bare Minimum Workout: 1 set, 2 times per week (15–20 repetitions of each exercise per set). Approximately 20 minutes.

The Ideal Workout: 2 sets, 2–3 times per week (15–20 repetitions of each exercise per set). Approximately 30 minutes.

The Gung-Ho Workout: 3 sets, 3 times per week (15–20 repetitions of each exercise per set). Approximately 45 minutes.

Exercises for the Endo-Pear ●●●

SQUATS

(tones the buttocks, the front and the back of the thighs and the calves)

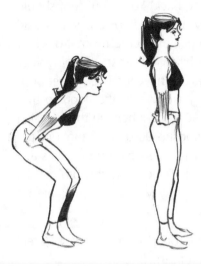

Stand with your feet hip-width apart, allowing for your natural turnout in the hips. Keeping the weight back on your heels, push your buttocks backward while reaching forward with your upper body. Your arms may be down or reaching out in front of you for balance. Bend until there is a 45- to 90-degree angle in your knees. Return to the starting position. Inhale on the way down and exhale on the way up.

SAFETY TIP: Make sure that you feel this exercise only in the thighs and the buttocks. If you feel strain in your knees, make sure that your weight is back on your heels and that your knees stay behind your toes at all times.

PLIES

(tones the buttocks, the front of the thighs, and the inner thighs)

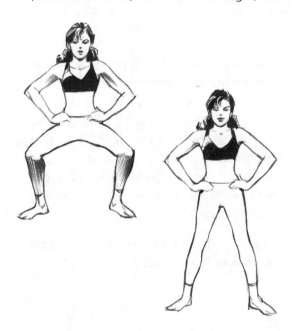

Stand with your legs turned out naturally from the hips. Your knees and toes should be in the same line. Bending at the knees and the hips, lower your buttocks straight down toward the floor until your knees are at a 45-degree angle. Slowly straighten your legs and return to the starting position. Exhale as you straighten your legs and inhale as you bend them.

SAFETY TIP: Make sure that you feel the work in the thighs and the buttocks and not in the knees. If you feel any discomfort in the knees, make sure that you aren't going down too far and that your knees and feet are in the same line.

STATIONARY LUNGES

(tones the buttocks and the front and the back of the thighs)

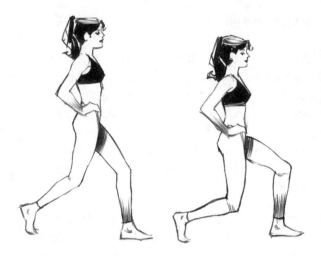

Stand with your right leg forward and your left leg back. Your front foot should be flat down on the floor, and you should be on the ball of your left foot. Your feet should be hip-width apart. Keeping your right knee behind your toes, lower your body straight down to the floor, so that there is a 90-degree bend in the front leg and an opposite 90-degree angle in the back leg. Then raise back up to the starting position. Repeat on the other side. Inhale on the way down and exhale on the way up

SAFETY TIP: Keep the front knee back behind the toes. Make sure that you feel the work in the thighs and the buttocks and not in the knees.

LYING LEG CIRCLES

(tones the outer thighs)

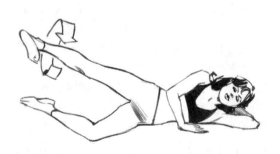

Lie on your right side on a mat or a padded surface with your forearm down. Your torso should be straight and your knees bent so that your upper thigh is at a 45-degree angle with your body. Raise your right leg so that the right knee is on top of the left one and "draw" a 12-inch circle in the air with your right heel. Repeat on the other side. Breathe evenly throughout.

SAFETY TIP: Keep your abdominals drawn in at all times. Keep the weight on your forearm and try to stay balanced on your hip. Do not lean backward.

BALL SQUEEZES

(tones the inner thighs, the buttocks, and the back of the legs)

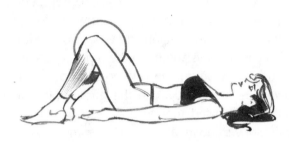

Lie on your back on a mat or a padded surface with your knees bent and your feet flat on the floor. Place a 6- to 10-inch ball between your inner thighs in a comfortable spot. Lift your buttocks off the floor and squeeze your inner thighs together so that they squeeze the ball tightly. Contract and lift your buttocks several inches off the floor. Hold this position for a second, then slowly lower the ball down without completely relaxing. Repeat. Exhale as you lift and inhale as you lower.

PERFORMANCE TIP: You may substitute a very firm throw pillow or a couch bolster for the ball.

PUSH-UPS

(tones the chest, the shoulders, and the back of the upper arms)

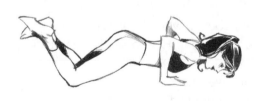

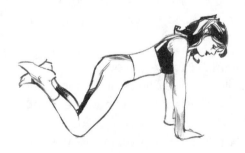

Kneel on a mat or a padded surface and place your hands on the floor about 6 to 8 inches away from your body, with your fingertips forward. Your hands should align with the nipple line of your chest. With a controlled motion, slowly bend your elbows and lower your chest toward the ground. Stop when your elbow is at a 90-degree bend and press back up to the starting position. Exhale as you push up and inhale as you lower yourself down.

SAFETY TIP: Don't lock your elbows out at the top or use momentum.

PERFORMANCE TIP: Keep your back flat, your abdominals tight, and your buttocks squeezed together. Keep the weight on the heels of your hands.

ROWS

(tones the back muscles and the front of the upper arms)

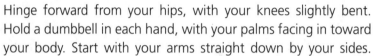

Hinge forward from your hips, with your knees slightly bent. Hold a dumbbell in each hand, with your palms facing in toward your body. Start with your arms straight down by your sides. Bend your elbows and bring the weights straight up until they are in line with your torso. Slowly lower the weights back to the starting position with a controlled motion. Exhale as you bend your elbows and inhale as you lower the weights back to the starting position.

SAFETY TIP: Protect your back by keeping your spine straight while at a 45-degree angle with the floor. Keep your abdominals drawn in tight and slightly bend your knees. If you cannot keep your back from rounding, place one hand on a chair back for support and perform the exercise one arm at a time.

PULLOVERS

(tones the chest, the back muscles, and the back of the upper arms)

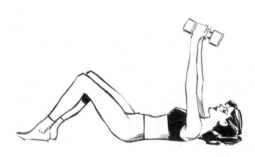

Lie on your back with your knees bent and your feet flat on the floor. Hold a single dumbbell securely with both hands over your belly button. Slowly lower the weight down toward the floor with a controlled motion, and return to the starting position. Inhale as you lower the weight over your head and exhale as you return to the starting position.

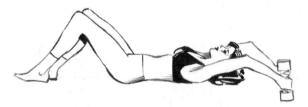

SAFETY TIP: Keep your abdominals pulled in at all times and your lower back pressed down into the floor. Lower the weight slowly and with a controlled motion. Don't use momentum in either direction.

DIPS

(tones the back of the upper arms)

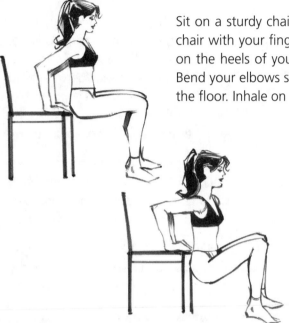

Sit on a sturdy chair and place your hands on the seat of the chair with your fingertips facing forward. Keeping the weight on the heels of your hands, slide your buttocks off the chair. Bend your elbows slightly and lower your body weight toward the floor. Inhale on the way down and exhale on the way up.

SAFETY TIP: Bend your elbows only to a 45- to 90-degree angle, not more. Try to keep your chest open and your shoulders back. Make sure you feel the work in the back of the upper arms and not in the front of your shoulders. If you feel any shoulder discomfort, make the movement less deep.

PERFORMANCE TIP: Keep your buttocks very close to the chair at all times.

BICEP CURLS

(tones the front of the upper arms)

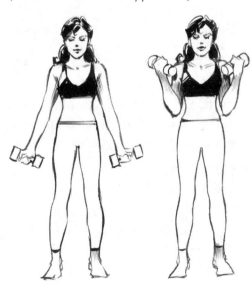

Stand straight and tall, holding a dumbbell in each hand. Your knees should be slightly bent, with your abdominals pulled in, your chest lifted, and your shoulders back. Bending only from the elbows, raise the weights up toward your shoulders. Keep your elbows in toward your side; don't use momentum in the arms. Don't move your back. Exhale as you raise the weights up and inhale as you lower them back down.

PERFORMANCE TIP: Be sure to lower the weights back to the starting position slowly and with a controlled motion.

REVERSE FLYS

(tones the middle of the back and the back of the shoulders)

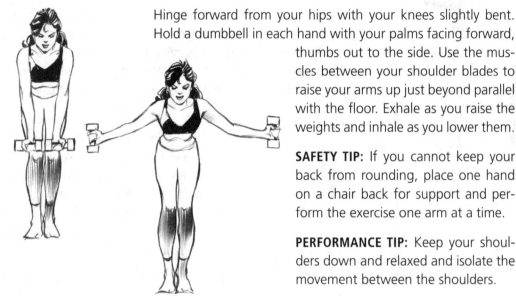

Hinge forward from your hips with your knees slightly bent. Hold a dumbbell in each hand with your palms facing forward, thumbs out to the side. Use the muscles between your shoulder blades to raise your arms up just beyond parallel with the floor. Exhale as you raise the weights and inhale as you lower them.

SAFETY TIP: If you cannot keep your back from rounding, place one hand on a chair back for support and perform the exercise one arm at a time.

PERFORMANCE TIP: Keep your shoulders down and relaxed and isolate the movement between the shoulders.

LOWER-BACK LIFTS

(tones the muscles that run along the spine)

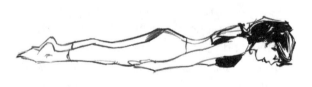

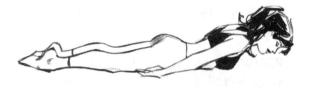

Lie facedown on a mat or a padded surface, with your arms alongside your body, palms facing upward. Keep the area from your waist down pressed into the floor and lift from the waist up, just a few inches off the ground. Exhale as you lift and inhale as you lower.

SAFETY TIP: Be sure to look straight down at the floor to protect your neck. Don't come up too high; you should feel only the muscles alongside your spine working, without any pinching or discomfort at all.

CURL-UPS

(tones the abdominals)

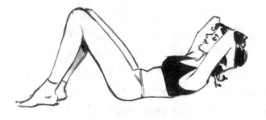

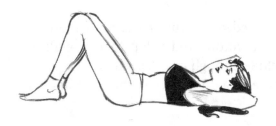

Lie on your back on a mat or a padded surface, with your knees bent and your feet flat on the floor. Lace your fingers behind your head. Keeping your head heavy in your hands, lift your upper body up so that your head, neck, and shoulders come off the mat. Then slowly lower them down, without completely relaxing, and repeat. Exhale as you lift up and inhale as you lower down.

SAFETY TIP: Keep your abdominals pulled in and your lower back pressed down into the floor.

PERFORMANCE TIP: If you find it difficult to keep your lower back pressed down, try lifting your toes off the floor while keeping the heels down.

BICYCLES

(tones abdominals)

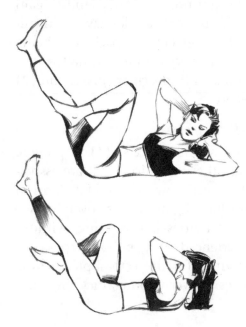

Lie on your back on a mat or a padded surface with your legs lifted at a 45-degree angle. Draw your right knee in toward your chest as you bring your left armpit toward your right knee. Then return to the starting position, and draw your left knee toward your chest and your right armpit toward your knee. Alternate between these two positions almost as if you were riding on a bicycle.

PERFORMANCE TIP: Be sure to keep your abdominals drawn in and your lower back pressed down into the floor

SAFETY TIP: Do only as many of these as you can without feeling any strain in your neck or lower back.

Paula, the Ecto-Apple ●●●

Every woman in the gym wants to look like Paula. Slender all over, with long, thin legs, Paula looks like a model because she is one. When Paula came to me for a consultation, she told me that she wanted to have a rear end like J-Lo's and finally get rid of her "gut." While I stared incredulously at her flawless body, she lifted up her shirt to show me her midsection. Though Paula was hardly overweight, she actually did have a soft midsection, relative to the rest of her body. Paula told me that she had never worked out consistently before and was looking for a program to tone her abdominals and add more womanly curves to her lower body.

Because Paula is an ecto-apple, she needed to focus on resistance training with heavier weights and fewer repetitions to develop more overall muscularity. She also needed to include enough cardiovascular exercise to reduce the only stubborn fat storage area on her body—her midriff.

Training the Ecto-Apple Body Type

Like her ecto-pear counterpart, the typical ecto-apple is blessed with a speedy metabolism. Naturally slender, with hardly any curves at all, the ecto-apple has the leanest appearance of all the body types.

While ecto-apples rarely have a weight problem, they tend to gain body fat exclusively in the midsection. Also, ecto-apples have a difficult time increasing muscle mass and often perceive themselves as being "too bony" or having a "boy's body." The ecto-apple is usually interested in (1) filling out her proportions with muscular curves, and (2) reducing body fat in the abdominal area.

Cardiovascular Fitness Guidelines for the Ecto-Apple

Ecto-apples need just enough cardiovascular exercise (1) to provide protection against heart disease and other conditions that are associated with the apple shape, and (2) to keep down visceral fat stores in the midsection. Because ecto-apples have lighter frames overall, they can often engage in higher-impact activities like running, without incurring the injuries frequently experienced by larger body types.

The best choices of aerobic activities for the ecto-apple include jogging, multi-impact aerobics classes, power walking, bicycling, and swimming.

The Fit + Female Cardio Rx for the Ecto-Apple

All three workout levels for the ecto-apple ("bare-minimum," "ideal," and "gung-ho") will have the same 20 minutes of cardiovascular exercise 3 times per week at lower to moderate intensities.

Muscular Fitness Guidelines for the Ecto-Apple

The foundation of the ecto-apple training program is weight workouts with heavier weight loads and fewer repetitions (6–12 repetitions per set) to fill out her proportions with increased muscularity.

The Fit + Female Muscular Fitness Rx for the Ecto-Apple

The Bare Minimum Workout: 1 set, 2 times per week (6–12 repetitions of each exercise per set). Approximately 20 minutes.

The Ideal Workout: 2 sets, 2–3 times per week (6–12 repetitions of each exercise per set). Approximately 30–40 minutes.

The Gung-Ho Workout: 3 sets, 3 times per week (6–12 repetitions of each exercise per set). Approximately 1 hour.

Exercises for the Ecto-Apple ●●○

STEP-UPS

(tones the buttocks, the front and the back of the thighs, and the calves)

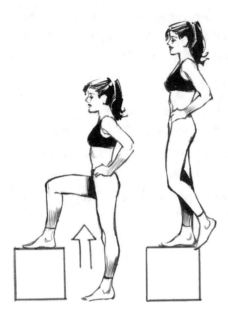

Stand with one foot on a sturdy bench or a step that's 6 to 12 inches high (the right step height for you should cause a 90-degree bend at your knee when you place your foot on it). Put all of your body weight on that same foot and, using your buttocks and thigh muscles, pull your body weight up on the step so that the other foot touches the step as well. Slowly lower yourself back to the starting position with a controlled motion. Exhale on the way up and inhale on the way down.

SAFETY TIP: Make sure that you feel this exercise only in the thighs and the buttocks. If you feel strain in your knees, make sure that your weight is back on your heels and that your knees stay behind your toes at all times.

PERFORMANCE TIP: Be sure not to use momentum to pull yourself up or lower yourself back down.

TOUCH-DOWNS

(tones the buttocks and the entire thigh)

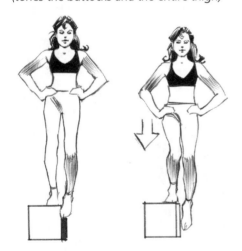

Stand with one foot on a sturdy stool or step. Contracting all of the muscles of the leg on the stool, slowly lower the other leg toward the floor as far as you can with a controlled motion. Then raise up to the starting position. Inhale as you lower toward the floor and exhale as you come back up.

SAFETY TIP: If you find this exercise too difficult at first, wait a few weeks until you develop more strength in your legs and then try the movement with a small range of motion.

SQUAT-SIDE LEG LIFTS

(tones the buttocks, the front and the back of the thighs, and the outer thighs)

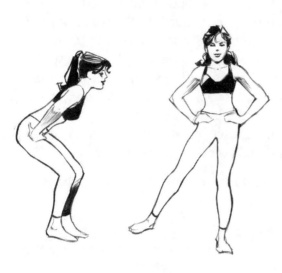

Stand with your feet hip-width apart, toes forward, allowing for your natural turnout in the hips. Bend your knees and push your buttocks backward, keeping the weight on your heels. As you return to the starting position, lift one leg out to the side, keeping the toes pointed forward. Raise the side of the leg toward the ceiling. Lower the leg back down and repeat, this time lifting the other leg. Exhale as you lift the leg and inhale as you lower it.

PERFORMANCE TIP: Keep your torso upright and try not to lean over to the opposite side as much as possible.

BALL SQUEEZES

(tones the inner thighs, the buttocks, and the back of the legs)

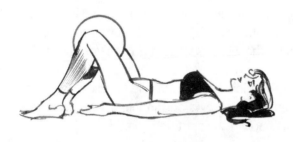

Lie on your back on a mat or a padded surface with your knees bent and your feet flat on the floor. Place a 6- to 10-inch ball between your inner thighs in a comfortable spot. Lift your buttocks off the floor and squeeze your inner thighs together so that they squeeze the ball tightly. Contract and lift your buttocks several inches off the floor. Hold this position for a second, then slowly lower the ball down without completely relaxing. Repeat. Exhale as you lift and inhale as you lower.

PERFORMANCE TIP: You may substitute a very firm throw pillow or a couch bolster for the ball.

PUSH-UPS

(tones the chest, the shoulders, and the back of the upper arms)

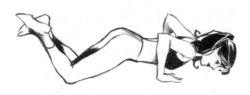

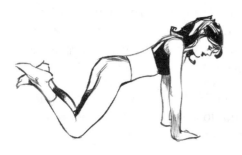

Kneel on a mat or a padded surface and place your hands on the floor about 6 to 8 inches away from your body, with your fingertips forward. Your hands should align with the nipple line of your chest. With a controlled motion, slowly bend your elbows and lower your chest toward the ground. Stop when the elbow is at a 90-degree bend, and press back up to the starting position. Exhale as you push up and inhale as you lower yourself down.

SAFETY TIP: Don't lock your elbows out at the top or use momentum.

PERFORMANCE TIP: Keep your back flat, your abdominals tight, and your buttocks squeezed together. Keep the weight on the heels of your hands.

ROWS

(tones the back muscles and the front of the upper arms)

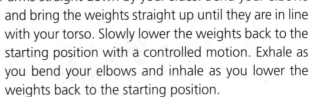

Hinge forward from your hips, with your knees slightly bent. Hold a dumbbell in each hand, with your palms facing in toward your body. Start with your arms straight down by your sides. Bend your elbows and bring the weights straight up until they are in line with your torso. Slowly lower the weights back to the starting position with a controlled motion. Exhale as you bend your elbows and inhale as you lower the weights back to the starting position.

SAFETY TIP: Protect your back by keeping your spine straight while at a 45-degree angle with the floor. Keep your abdominals drawn in tight and slightly bend your knees. If you cannot keep your back from rounding, place one hand on a chair back for support and perform the exercise one arm at a time.

PULLOVERS

(tones the chest, the back muscles, and the back of the upper arms)

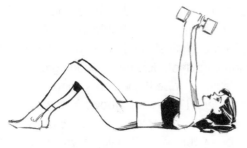

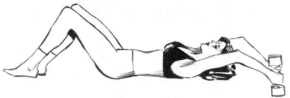

Lie on your back with your knees bent and your feet flat on the floor. Hold a single dumbbell securely with both hands over your belly button. Slowly lower the weight down toward the floor with a controlled motion and return to the starting position. Inhale as you lower the weight over your head and exhale as you return it to the starting position.

SAFETY TIP: Keep your abdominals pulled in at all times and your lower back pressed down into the floor. Lower the weight slowly and with a controlled motion. Don't use momentum in either direction.

DIPS

(tones the back of the upper arms)

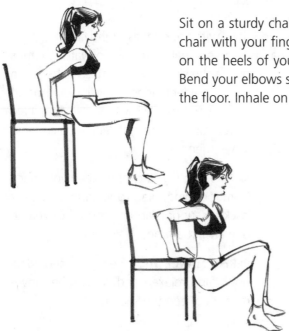

Sit on a sturdy chair and place your hands on the seat of the chair with your fingertips facing forward. Keeping the weight on the heels of your hands, slide your buttocks off the chair. Bend your elbows slightly and lower your body weight toward the floor. Inhale on the way down and exhale on the way up.

SAFETY TIP: Bend your elbows only to a 45- to 90-degree angle, not more. Try to keep your chest open and your shoulders back. Make sure you feel the work in the back of the upper arms and not in the front of your shoulders. If you feel any shoulder discomfort, make the movement less deep.

PERFORMANCE TIP: Keep your buttocks very close to the chair at all times.

BICEP CURLS

(tones the front of the upper arms)

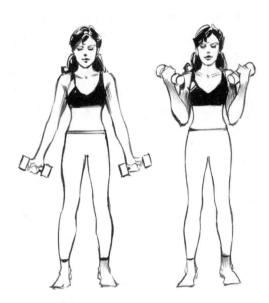

Stand straight and tall, holding a dumbbell in each hand. Your knees should be slightly bent, your abdominals pulled in, your chest lifted, and your shoulders back. Bending only from the elbows, raise the weights up toward your shoulders. Keep your elbows in toward your side; don't use momentum in the arms. Don't move your back. Exhale as you raise the weights up and inhale as you lower them back down.

PERFORMANCE TIP: Be sure to lower the weights back to the starting position slowly and with a controlled motion.

REVERSE FLYS

(tones the middle of the back and the back of the shoulders)

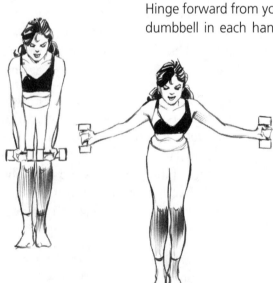

Hinge forward from your hips with your knees slightly bent. Hold a dumbbell in each hand with your palms facing forward, thumbs out to the side. Use the muscles between your shoulder blades to raise your arms up just beyond parallel with the floor. Exhale as you raise the weights and inhale as you lower them.

SAFETY TIP: If you cannot keep your back from rounding, place one hand on a chair back for support and perform the exercise one arm at a time.

PERFORMANCE TIP: Keep your shoulders down and relaxed and isolate the movement between the shoulders.

LOWER-BACK LIFTS

(tones the muscles that run along the spine)

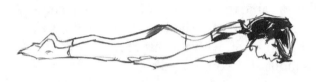

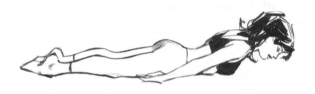

Lie facedown on a mat or a padded surface, with your arms alongside your body, palms facing upward. Keep the area from your waist down pressed into the floor and lift from the waist up, just a few inches off the ground. Exhale as you lift and inhale as you lower.

SAFETY TIP: Be sure to look straight down at the floor to protect your neck. Don't come up too high; you should feel only the muscles alongside your spine working, without any pinching or discomfort at all.

ABDOMINAL CRUNCHES*

(tones the abdominals)

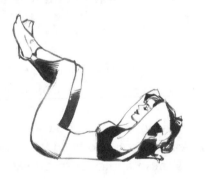

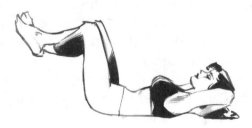

Lie on your back with your knees bent, your feet crossed at the ankles, and your hands placed gently behind your head. Lift your upper body and your legs up and in toward the center of your body at the same time. Then slowly lower them back to the starting position. Exhale as you bend your body and inhale as you lower back to the starting position.

SAFETY TIP: Keep your abdominals pulled in tight throughout the movement and your lower back pressed down into the floor. Keep your neck relaxed by letting the weight of your head fall into your hands.

Eva, the Meso-Apple ●●●

When people see Eva's legs, they assume she works out—a lot. Cut and toned, without an ounce of body fat, Eva's legs look as if she spends hours in the gym. The truth is that except for the occasional brisk walk, Eva hardly works out at all. Eva came to me to see if I could help similarly define her waistline. She told me that she has always had a soft stomach that seemed out of proportion with the rest of her body.

I told Eva that as a meso-apple, she would need some moderate cardiovascular exercise and torso toning to help whittle her waist. However, because of her considerable natural muscle tone in the rest of her body, Eva would need minimal resistance training to maintain a sculpted look in the rest of her body.

Training the Meso-Apple Body Type

The meso-apple has well-developed, sinewy legs and very little body fat in the upper body. This body type never gains weight (or bulk) in the lower body. Even at their most slender, though, meso-apples have a hard time developing muscular definition in their abdominals. Some meso-apples are also prone to gaining weight in the breasts, as well as in the waist. Fortunately, cardiovascular workouts and resistance training, with a focus on core exercises, can go a long way toward making this body type a true athletic inspiration.

Cardiovascular Fitness Guidelines for the Meso-Apple

Many meso-apples are obsessed with crunches and sit-ups because they mistakenly believe that endless ab exercises are the key to achieving a wasp waist. However, for the meso-apple, cardiovascular workouts are actually the most important factor in developing a "six-pack." It is proper aerobic conditioning that removes the excess body fat from any body part, regardless of location. Unless meso-apples burn off excess fat tissue from their torsos, even the most toned muscles will remain obscured under an extra layer of padding. Like ecto-apples, meso-apples can usually choose from a wide variety of cardiovascular workouts, including those with higher impact.

The best choices of aerobic activities for the meso-apple include jogging, multi-impact aerobics classes, power walking, kickboxing, and bicycling.

The Fit + Female Cardio Rx for the Meso-Apple

> The Bare Minimum Workout: 30 minutes, 3 times per week
>
> The Ideal Workout: 30–45 minutes, 3–5 times per week
>
> The Gung-Ho Workout: 45–60 minutes, 3–5 times per week

Muscular Fitness Guidelines for the Meso-Apple

The foundation of the meso-apple training program will focus on moderate weights with moderate repetitions (12–15 repetitions of each exercise per set) and concentrated torso toning.

The Fit + Female Muscular Fitness Rx for the Meso-Apple

> The Bare Minimum Workout: 1 set, 2 times per week (12–15 repetitions of each exercise per set). Approximately 20 minutes. Plus the torso exercises (indicated with an *) 3 times per week. Approximately 5 minutes.
>
> The Ideal Workout: 2 sets, 2 times per week (12–15 repetitions of each exercise per set). Approximately 30 minutes. Plus the torso exercises (indicated with an *) 3–5 times per week. Approximately 5 minutes.
>
> The Gung-Ho Workout: 3 sets, 2 times per week (12–15 repetitions of each exercise per set). Approximately 40 minutes. Plus the torso exercises (indicated with an *) 5 times per week. Approximately 5 minutes.

Exercises for the Meso-Apple ●●●

PLIES

(tones the buttocks, the front of the thighs, and the inner thighs)

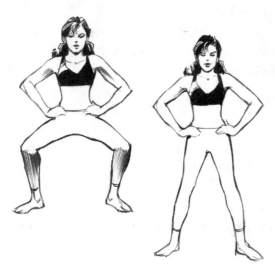

Stand with your legs turned out naturally from the hips. Your knees and toes should be in the same line. Bending at the knees and the hips, lower your buttocks straight down toward the floor until your knees are at a 45-degree angle. Slowly straighten your legs and return to the starting position. Exhale as you straighten your legs and inhale as you bend them

SAFETY TIP: Make sure that you feel the work in the thighs and the buttocks and not in the knees. If you feel any discomfort in the knees, make sure that you aren't going down too far and that your knees and feet are in the same line.

SQUAT-SIDE LEG LIFTS

(tones the buttocks, the front and back of the thighs, and the outer thighs)

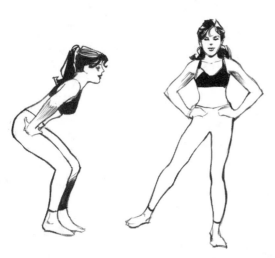

Stand with your feet hip-width apart, toes forward, allowing for your natural turnout in the hips. Bend your knees and push your buttocks backward, keeping the weight on your heels. As you return to the starting position, lift one leg out to the side, keeping the toes pointed forward. Raise the side of the leg toward the ceiling. Lower the leg back down and repeat, this time lifting the other leg. Exhale as you lift the leg and inhale as you lower it.

PERFORMANCE TIP: Keep your torso upright and try not to lean over to the opposite side as much as possible.

PUSH-UPS

(tones the chest, the shoulders, and the back of the upper arms)

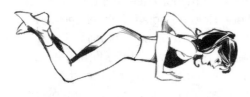

Kneel on a mat or a padded surface and place your hands on the floor about 6 to 8 inches away from your body, with your fingertips forward. Your hands should align with the nipple line of your chest. With a controlled motion, slowly bend your elbows and lower your chest toward the ground. Stop when the elbow is at a 90-degree bend and press back up to the starting position. Exhale as you push up and inhale as you lower yourself down.

SAFETY TIP: Don't lock your elbows out at the top or use momentum.

PERFORMANCE TIP: Keep your back flat, your abdominals tight, and your buttocks squeezed together. Keep the weight on the heels of your hands.

ROWS

(tones the back muscles and the front of the upper arms)

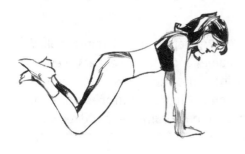

Hinge forward from your hips, with your knees slightly bent. Hold a dumbbell in each hand, with your palms facing in toward your body. Start with your arms straight down by your sides. Bend your elbows and bring the weights straight up until they are in line with your torso. Slowly lower the weights back to the starting position with a controlled motion. Exhale as you bend your elbows and inhale as you lower the weights back to the starting position.

SAFETY TIP: Protect your back by keeping your spine straight while at a 45-degree angle with the floor. Keep your abdominals drawn in tight and slightly bend your knees. If you cannot keep your back from rounding, place one hand on a chair back for support and perform the exercise one arm at a time.

PULLOVERS

(tones the chest, the back muscles, and the back of the upper arms)

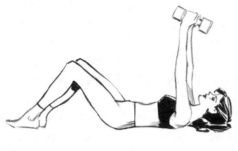

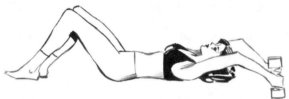

Lie on your back with your knees bent, your feet flat on the floor. Hold a single dumbbell securely with both hands over your belly button. Slowly lower the weight down toward the floor with a controlled motion, and return to the starting position. Inhale as you lower the weight over your head and exhale as you return it to the starting position.

SAFETY TIP: Keep your abdominals pulled in at all times and your lower back pressed down into the floor. Lower the weight slowly and with a controlled motion. Don't use momentum in either direction.

DIPS

(tones the back of the upper arms)

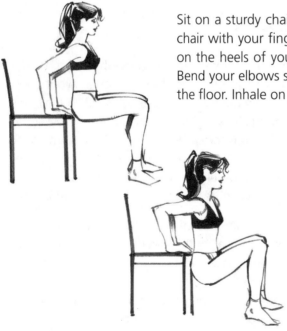

Sit on a sturdy chair and place your hands on the seat of the chair with your fingertips facing forward. Keeping the weight on the heels of your hands, slide your buttocks off the chair. Bend your elbows slightly and lower your body weight toward the floor. Inhale on the way down and exhale on the way up.

SAFETY TIP: Bend your elbows only to a 45- to 90-degree angle, not more. Try to keep your chest open and your shoulders back. Make sure you feel the work in the back of the upper arms and not in the front of your shoulders. If you feel any shoulder discomfort, make the movement less deep.

PERFORMANCE TIP: Keep your buttocks very close to the chair at all times.

BICEP CURLS

(tones the front of the upper arms)

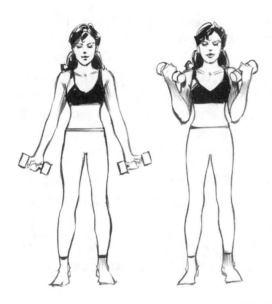

Stand straight and tall, holding a dumbbell in each hand. Your knees should be slightly bent, your abdominals pulled in, your chest lifted, and your shoulders back. Bending only from the elbows, raise the weights up toward your shoulders. Keep your elbows in toward your side; don't use momentum in your arms. Don't move your back. Exhale as you raise the weights up; inhale as you lower them back down.

PERFORMANCE TIP: Be sure to lower the weights back to the starting position slowly and with a controlled motion.

REVERSE FLYS

(tones the middle of the back and the back of the shoulders)

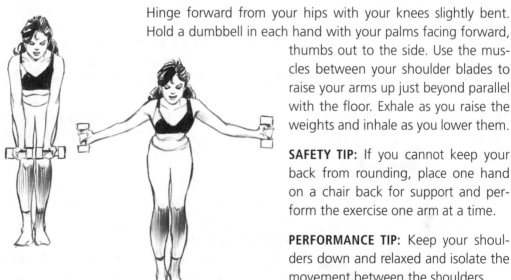

Hinge forward from your hips with your knees slightly bent. Hold a dumbbell in each hand with your palms facing forward, thumbs out to the side. Use the muscles between your shoulder blades to raise your arms up just beyond parallel with the floor. Exhale as you raise the weights and inhale as you lower them.

SAFETY TIP: If you cannot keep your back from rounding, place one hand on a chair back for support and perform the exercise one arm at a time.

PERFORMANCE TIP: Keep your shoulders down and relaxed and isolate the movement between the shoulders.

BICYCLES*

(tones the abdominals)

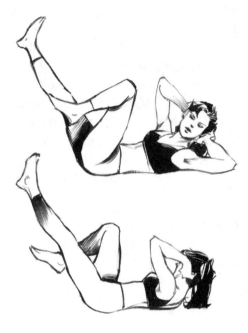

Lie on your back on a mat or a padded surface with your legs lifted at a 45-degree angle. Draw your right knee in toward your chest as you bring your left armpit toward your right knee. Then return to the starting position and draw your left knee toward your chest and your right armpit toward your knee. Alternate between these two positions, almost as if you were riding on a bicycle.

PERFORMANCE TIP: Be sure to keep your abdominals drawn in and your lower back pressed down into the floor.

SAFETY TIP: Do only as many of these as you can without feeling any strain in your neck or lower back.

ABDOMINAL CRUNCHES*

(tones the abdominals)

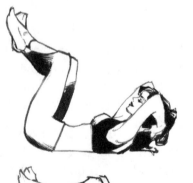

Lie on your back with your knees bent, your feet crossed at the ankles, and your hands placed gently behind your head. Lift your upper body and your legs up and in toward the center of your body at the same time. Then slowly lower them back to the starting position. Exhale as you bend your body and inhale as you lower back to the starting position.

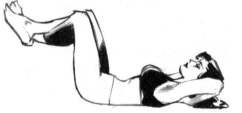

SAFETY TIP: Keep your abdominals pulled in tight throughout the movement and your lower back pressed down into the floor. Keep your neck relaxed by letting the weight of your head fall into your hands.

LATERAL FLEXION*

(tones the waist and the abdominals)

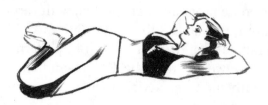

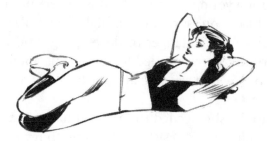

Lie on one side on a mat or a padded surface with your knees bent at a 45-degree angle out from your body. Your knees and feet should be touching. Place your hands behind your head, interlacing your fingers, and rotate your torso so that you are looking at the ceiling as much as is comfortable. Lift your head, neck, and shoulders off the mat as far as is comfortable and then lower them back down. Exhale as you lift and inhale as you lower. Repeat on the other side.

PERFORMANCE TIP: Concentrate on keeping your legs down and your waist pressed down to the floor as much as possible.

LOWER-BACK LIFTS*

(tones the muscles that run along the spine)

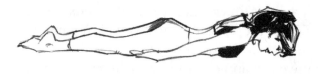

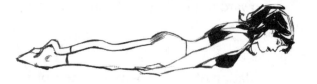

Lie facedown on a mat or a padded surface, with your arms alongside your body, palms facing upward. Keep the area from your waist down pressed into the floor and lift from the waist up, just a few inches off the ground. Exhale as you lift and inhale as you lower.

SAFETY TIP: Be sure to look straight down at the floor to protect your neck. Don't come up too high; you should feel only the muscles alongside your spine working without any pinching or discomfort at all.

Karen, the Endo-Apple ●●●

Karen was overweight, with a quintessential endo-apple shape—round and full through the upper body with slender legs. Since high school, Karen had tried one diet and exercise program after another, with varying degrees of success. The pattern was always the same. Karen would lose a few pounds and then gradually fall back into her old patterns, invariably gaining back all of the weight that she'd lost—and then some. Karen started to train with me after a visit to her physician revealed that her weight problems were more than skin deep.

The doctor told Karen that for a young woman, she was in very poor health. Tests revealed that her blood pressure was too high, her cholesterol was skyrocketing, and she was in danger of developing type 2 diabetes. The doctor's prescription: Karen needed to get serious about losing weight (and keeping it off) with a sensible approach to diet and exercise.

Because Karen is an endo-apple, she needed to focus on daily aerobic conditioning to burn off body fat and resistance training to rev up her sluggish metabolism. Most important, we needed to help Karen change her mindset about weight control, from one based on short-term fixes to one centered on a long-term plan of permanent wellness.

Training the Endo-Apple Body Type

The endo-apple tends to be full through the waist, the bust, and the upper arms but with well-defined legs and a small, even a flat, backside. It's very easy for this body type to gain weight through the midsection.

Of all the body types, endo-apples have the most variation, ranging from women of normal weight to those who are morbidly obese. Weight control is usually the endo-apple's primary challenge. A major source of frustration for this body type is that even at her thinnest, the typical endo-apple will never have a wasp waist. However, a sensible fitness program will go a long way toward improving her health and radically altering her proportions.

Cardiovascular Fitness Guidelines for the Endo-Apple

Cardiovascular training is the foundation of the endo-apple fitness program. There are "Three Ls" that the endo-apple must remember when selecting cardiovascular workouts. Specifically, endo-apples should focus on activities that are (1) of longer duration (to maximize calorie burn), (2) of lower intensity (to allow for longer workouts without fatigue), and (3) lower-impact (to prevent the injuries associated with jarring repetitive motions).

The best choices of aerobic activities for the endo-apple include power walking, bicycling, cross-country skiing, elliptical climbing machines, and low-impact aerobics classes.

The Fit + Female Cardio Rx for the Endo-Apple

The Bare Minimum Workout: 20–30 minutes, 3–5 times per week at 60 to 75 percent of the age-predicted heart rate max.

The Ideal Workout: 30–45 minutes, 3–5 times per week at 60 to 75 percent of the age-predicted heart rate max.

The Gung-Ho Workout: 45–60 minutes, 3–5 times per week at 60 to 75 percent of the age-predicted heart rate max.

Muscular Fitness Guidelines for the Endo-Apple

The endo-apple training program will focus on lighter weights with higher repetitions (15–20 repetitions per set) to sculpt and define the upper body, plus concentrated torso toning. Resistance training is particularly important for the endo-apple because it increases muscle tissue. Having more muscle tone elevates resting metabolism and promotes weight control.

The Fit + Female Muscular Fitness Rx for the Endo-Apple

The Bare Minimum Workout: 1 set, 2 times per week (15–20 repetitions of each exercise per set). Approximately 25 minutes. Plus the torso exercises (indicated with an *) 3 times per week. Approximately 5 minutes.

The Ideal Workout: 2 sets, 2 times per week (15–20 repetitions of each exercise per set). Approximately 35 minutes. Plus the torso exercises (indicated with an *) 3–5 times per week. Approximately 5 minutes.

The Gung-Ho Workout: 3 sets, 2 times per week (15–20 repetitions of each exercise per set). Approximately 45 minutes. Plus the torso exercises (indicated with an *) 5 times per week. Approximately 5 minutes.

Exercises for the Endo-Apple ●●●

PLIES

(tones the buttocks, the front of the thighs, and the inner thighs)

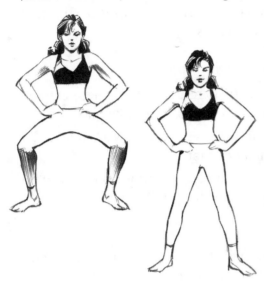

Stand with your legs turned out naturally from the hips. Your knees and toes should be in the same line. Bending at the knees and the hips, lower your buttocks straight down toward the floor until the knees are at a 45-degree angle. Slowly straighten your legs and return to the starting position. Exhale as you straighten your legs and inhale and you bend them.

SAFETY TIP: Make sure that you feel the work in the thighs and the buttocks and not in the knees. If you feel any discomfort in the knees, make sure that you aren't going down too far and that your knees and feet are in the same line.

SQUAT-SIDE LEG LIFTS

(tones the buttocks, the front and the back of the thighs, and the outer thighs)

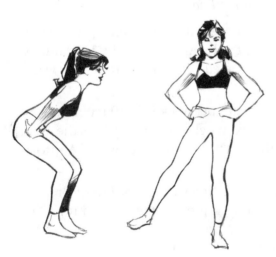

Stand with your feet hip-width apart, toes forward, allowing for your natural turnout in the hips. Bend your knees and push your buttocks backward, keeping the weight on your heels. As you return to the starting position, lift one leg out to the side, keeping the toes pointed forward. Raise the side of the leg toward the ceiling. Lower the leg back down and repeat, this time lifting the other leg. Exhale as you lift the leg and inhale as you lower it.

PERFORMANCE TIP: Keep your torso upright, and try not to lean over to the opposite side as much as possible.

PUSH-UPS

(tones the chest, the shoulders, and the back of the upper arms)

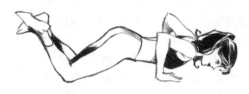

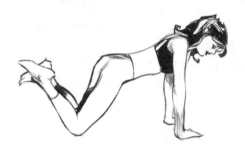

Kneel on a mat or a padded surface, and place your hands on the floor about 6 to 8 inches away from your body, with your fingertips forward. Your hands should align with the nipple line of your chest. With a controlled motion, slowly bend your elbows and lower your chest toward the ground. Stop when each elbow is at a 90-degree bend and then press back up to the starting position. Exhale as you push up and inhale as you lower yourself down.

SAFETY TIP: Don't lock your elbows out at the top or use momentum.

PERFORMANCE TIP: Keep your back flat, your abdominals tight, and your buttocks squeezed together. Keep the weight on the heels of your hands.

ROWS

(tones the back muscles and the front of the upper arms)

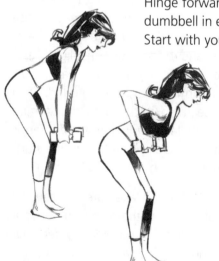

Hinge forward from your hips, with your knees slightly bent. Hold a dumbbell in each hand, with your palms facing in toward your body. Start with your arms straight down by your sides. Bend your elbows and bring the weights straight up until they are in line with your torso. Slowly lower the weights back to the starting position with a controlled motion. Exhale as you bend your elbows and inhale as you lower the weights back to the starting position.

SAFETY TIP: Protect your back by keeping your spine straight while at a 45-degree angle with the floor. Keep your abdominals drawn in tight and slightly bend your knees. If you cannot keep your back from rounding, place one hand on a chair back for support and perform the exercise one arm at a time.

PULLOVERS

(tones the chest, the back muscles, and the back of the upper arms)

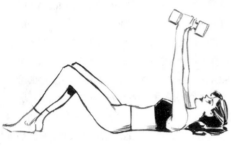

Lie on your back with your knees bent, your feet flat on the floor. Hold a single dumbbell securely with both hands over your belly button. Slowly lower the weight down toward the floor with a controlled motion and return it to the starting position. Inhale as you lower the weight over your head and exhale as you return it to the starting position.

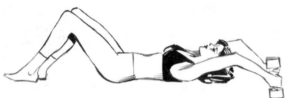

SAFETY TIP: Keep your abdominals pulled in at all times and your lower back pressed down into the floor. Lower the weight slowly and with a controlled motion. Don't use momentum in either direction.

FLYS

(tones the chest muscles, the front of the shoulders, and the front of the upper arms)

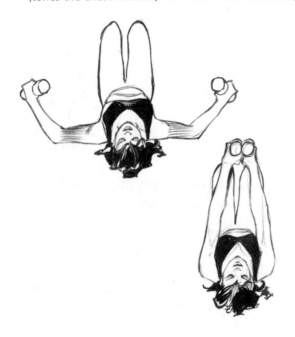

Lie on your back on a mat or a padded surface with your knees bent, your feet flat on the floor. Hold dumbbells in both hands with your hands resting on your stomach. Raise your arms straight up over the nipple line of your chest and round your arms slightly as if you were hugging a giant beach ball. Slowly lower your arms down to the ground. Then slowly raise them back up to the starting position. Inhale as you lower your arms down and exhale as you return to the starting position.

PERFORMANCE TIP: Make sure to keep the weights directly over the nipple line of your chest throughout the movement. Keep your shoulders down and relaxed at all times.

TRICEP KICKBACKS

(tones the back of the upper arms)

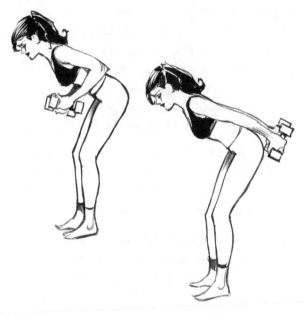

Stand with your feet together, knees bent slightly, and holding a 2- to 5-pound dumbbell in each hand. Bend forward from your hips, with your abdominals pulled in tightly, and your back straight but at a 45-degree angle with your hips. Lift your upper arms and pin them in close to your sides, turn your hands so that the dumbbells face in toward your body. Using the muscles in the back of your upper arms, lift the weights until your elbows are straight and lower them back down. Repeat. Exhale as you straighten your arms and inhale as you lower them.

PERFORMANCE TIP: Straighten the elbows, but don't lock them out.

BICEP CURLS

(tones the front of the upper arms)

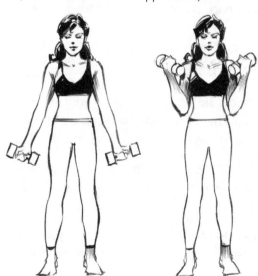

Stand straight and tall, holding a dumbbell in each hand. Your knees should be slightly bent, with your abdominals pulled in, your chest lifted, and your shoulders back. Bending only from the elbows, raise the weights up toward your shoulders. Keep your elbows in toward your side; don't use momentum in the arms. Don't move your back. Exhale as you raise the weights up and inhale as you lower them back down.

PERFORMANCE TIP: Be sure to lower the weights back to the starting position slowly and with a controlled motion.

REVERSE FLYS

(tones the middle of the back and the back of the shoulders)

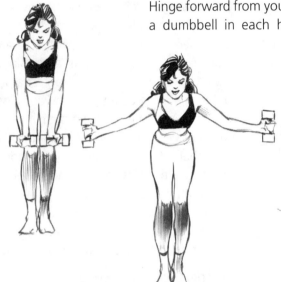

Hinge forward from your hips with your knees slightly bent. Hold a dumbbell in each hand with your palms facing forward, thumbs out to the side. Use the muscles between your shoulder blades to raise your arms up just beyond parallel with the floor. Exhale as you raise the weights and inhale as you lower them.

SAFETY TIP: If you cannot keep your back from rounding, place one hand on a chair back for support and perform the exercise one arm at a time.

PERFORMANCE TIP: Keep your shoulders down and relaxed and isolate the movement between the shoulders.

BICYCLES*

(tones the abdominals)

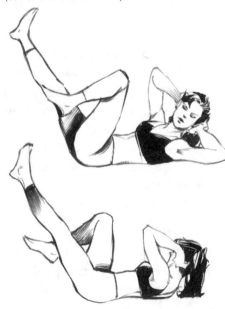

Lie on your back on a mat or a padded surface with your legs lifted at a 45-degree angle. Draw your right knee in toward your chest as you bring your left armpit toward your right knee. Then return to the starting position, and draw your left knee toward your chest and your right armpit toward your knee. Alternate between these two positions, almost as if you were riding on a bicycle.

PERFORMANCE TIP: Be sure to keep your abdominals drawn in and your lower back pressed down into the floor.

SAFETY TIP: Do only as many of these as you can without feeling any strain in your neck or lower back.

ABDOMINAL CRUNCHES*

(tones the abdominals)

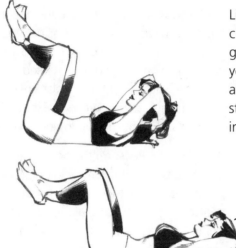

Lie on your back with your knees bent, your feet crossed at the ankles, and your hands placed gently behind your head. Lift your upper body and your legs up and in toward the center of your body at the same time. Then slowly lower back to the starting position. Exhale as you bend your body and inhale as you lower back to the starting position.

SAFETY TIP: Keep your abdominals pulled in tight throughout the movement and your lower back pressed down into the floor. Keep your neck relaxed by letting the weight of your head fall into your hands.

LATERAL FLEXION*

(tones the waist and the abdominals)

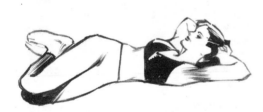

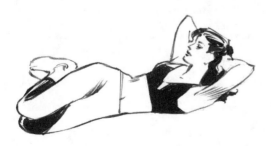

Lie on one side on a mat or a padded surface with your knees bent at a 45-degree angle out from your body. Your knees and feet should be touching. Place your hands behind your head, interlacing your fingers, and rotate your torso so that you are looking at the ceiling as much as is comfortable. Lift your head, neck, and shoulders off the mat as far as is comfortable and then lower them back down. Exhale as you lift and inhale as you lower. Repeat on the other side.

PERFORMANCE TIP: Concentrate on keeping your legs down and your waist pressed down to the floor as much as possible.

LOWER-BACK LIFTS*

(tones the muscles that run along the spine)

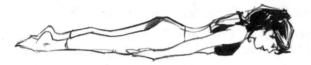

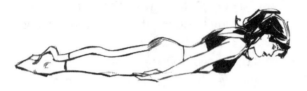

Lie facedown on a mat or a padded surface, with your arms alongside your body, palms facing upward. Keep the area from your waist down pressed into the floor and lift from the waist up, just a few inches off the ground. Exhale as you lift and inhale as you lower.

SAFETY TIP: Be sure to look straight down at the floor to protect your neck. Don't come up too high; you should feel only the muscles alongside your spine working, without any pinching or discomfort at all.

8

how to put it all together: from warm-up to cool-down

As I mentioned in chapter 6, while there are crucial differences between each of the six workouts, some common elements are vital to all of them. Specifically, each workout (regardless of the body type) needs to begin with a warm-up and finish with a cool-down. This holds true for cardiovascular workouts and/or muscular fitness workouts. If you are going to move your muscles with exercise, you need to prepare them first with a warm-up and help them return to the resting state with a cool-down.

The Warm-Up ●●●

Warm-ups are one of the most commonly misunderstood components of a workout. In fact, a true warm-up is quite different from what most people imagine it to be.

Most people's notion of warming up consists of leaning against a fence post (or a wall) and holding a few stretches for a split second each, then rushing to start their workout.

Whenever I see this, I'm always tempted to walk up to the people and ask them (in all seriousness) just what they think they are accomplishing. The primary purpose of a warm-up is just that—to warm the body up. Standing still and stretching for a nanosecond does absolutely nothing to make that happen. This means that the stereotypical warm-ups that we see the weekend warrior doing before his run are actually more dangerous than beneficial.

For one thing, it's never a good idea to stretch a cold muscle. Cold muscles behave much in the way that cold taffy does; they aren't very pliable and will resist stretching to such a degree that they can actually tear.

For another, static stretches (the type of stretches where you don't move or bounce) need to be held for a minimum of fifteen seconds in order to be effective. This gives the muscles a chance to release and lengthen. Folks who do these brief pseudo warm-ups would actually be better off doing nothing at all.

Ideally, a properly structured warm-up will

Increase blood flow to the working muscles

Prepare the muscle fibers to contract

Increase oxygen delivery to the muscles

Increase the delivery of blood sugar to fuel the brain and the muscles

Warm up the joints

Allow the central nervous system (the brain and the nerves) to ready the body for movement

Prepare the cardiovascular system for the increased intensity of exercise

Provide increased blood supply to the heart muscle itself

In addition, it's not known for sure but scientists also believe that warm-ups may improve athletic performance and prevent muscle soreness, muscle strains to the ligaments, and the tearing of muscle fibers or tendons.

The easiest and most effective way to warm up the body is to begin by moving the larger muscles first. For most activities, this can be accomplished simply by doing a slower-pace, lower-intensity version of the activity you are about to do. You want to do large movements in a full and fluid range of motion. This kind of activity improves blood flow to the muscles that will be used during the exercises to follow. Improved blood flow raises muscle temperature and decreases muscle tension. In addition, joint movement increases the quality (and the quantity) of the fluid that lubricates joints, known as the synovial fluid.

A good indication that the warm-up is working is that the body temperature increases about 1 degree Fahrenheit. Since most of us don't walk around with a thermometer in our back pockets, though, an easier way to measure this is simply having the feeling that you want to shed a layer of workout gear.

This brings up another important point. When you exercise, you should plan on wearing several layers of clothing. For example: a first layer of a jogging bra and leggings, with a T-shirt over the top, and perhaps a sweatshirt on top of that. By the time you've finished your warm-up, you should feel warm enough that you want to remove (at least) the first layer of clothing. That is why warm-ups will always take more time in colder environments and less time in hotter environments.

Here are some other important points about warm-ups to keep in mind. A warm-up should be a minimum of 5 minutes. Depending on the person's age, injuries, fitness level, and individual differences, though, it may take as long as 20 minutes. Pregnant women, older women, and those with joint and muscle problems (such as arthritis) will also need longer warm-ups. Most of these women should plan on doing a minimum of 15 minutes before their workouts. Also, though it's important to get warm from the warm-up, it's just as crucial not to get overheated. You should dress in layers in order to allow air circulation. This helps sweat to evaporate off the skin's surface and keeps the body cool. All pregnant women, especially those in their first trimester, should avoid getting overheated. A developing fetus cannot dissipate heat, and a dangerous increase in body temperature (from exercise or anything else) could result in a miscarriage. Pregnant women should always consult their physicians before beginning any exercise program.

Then, immediately after the body gets warm, it's a good idea to follow with some rhythmic, moving (but not bouncing) stretching for all of the major muscle groups. These range of motion (or dynamic stretching) moves simulate the kinds of movements that you do when exercising. They not only prepare the body for exercise; they may also protect against injuries.

Each of these movements should be done almost in slow motion.

They should be smooth and fluid movements, without any momentum. Start small, and as you continue to move, you should find that you can go a bit farther in the movement than before. However, it's important to be careful not to force any of the ranges of movement. You should be in control, and the movement should feel good at all times.

Step One: Getting Warm

If you have access to a cardiovascular machine (whether at home or at the gym), you can use that to warm yourself up. If you're exercising outside (doing a power walk, for example), you can do a lower-intensity version of your exercise. If you're biking, be sure that you're not pedaling fast and that there is very little to no tension during the warm-up. Whatever cardiovascular machine you choose (say, the elliptical machine, for example), just be sure to do the movement slowly, with little to no tension or inclines. The idea is simply to get moving gently and easily.

If you don't have access to a machine (or maybe it's a day when you just don't care to use one), the following series of movements will provide an effective total body warm-up.

It will probably take 5 to 10 minutes to do, but don't focus on doing this routine for a particular amount of time. Rather, focus on doing it long enough to feel considerably warmer by the time you're finished.

MARCHING IN PLACE WITH ARM PUMP

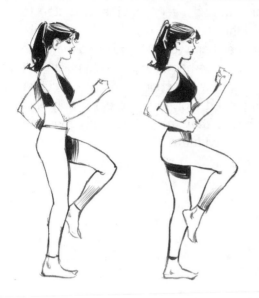

Standing straight and tall, begin marching in place while pumping your arms back and forth. Concentrate on smooth, full-body movements, lifting the knees as high as is comfortable.

THREE STEPS FORWARD WITH A KNEE/THREE STEPS BACK

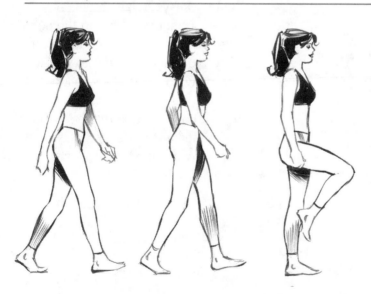

Take three steps forward, starting with the right foot. Step right, left, right, and then raise the left knee. Then step back with the left foot, stepping left, right, left, and raise the right knee.

STEP TOGETHER STEP TOUCH (MOVING LATERALLY)

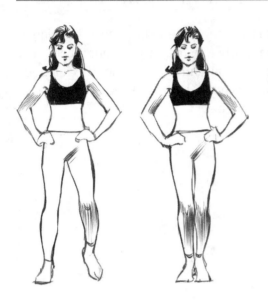

Begin with your feet together and step to the right about 24 inches with your right foot, then bring your left foot in so that both feet are together. Step out again with the right foot traveling right, then step together with the left foot, touching down only with the ball of the foot. Reverse directions and travel left with the left foot.

LOW-IMPACT SIDE JACKS

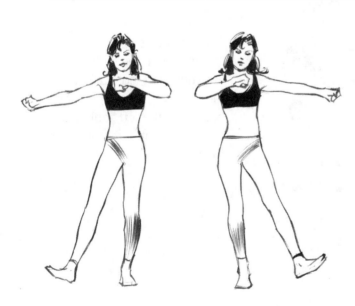

Stand with your feet together and place your right heel out to the right side of the room. Simultaneously punch your right arm out to the side and draw your left elbow backward as if you are about to shoot an arrow from a bow. Repeat on the left side and continue to alternate back and forth between the two positions.

ALTERNATING SIDE-TO-SIDE KNEES
WITH BOW AND ARROW ARMS

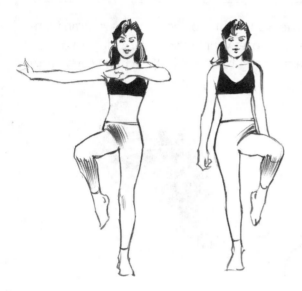

With the same bow-and-arrow arm movement that you used in the low-impact side jacks, alternate lifting your knees up and out to the side. Lift as high as possible, keeping your back straight at all times. Continue to alternate back and forth between the two positions.

ALTERNATING BUTT-KICKERS

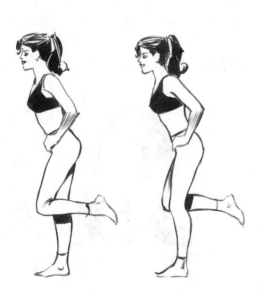

Step to the right with your right foot, while bending your left knee and bringing your left heel in toward your buttocks. Then step to the left with your left foot, while bending your right knee and bringing your right heel in toward your buttocks. Continue to alternate back and forth between the two positions.

THE LOOKY LOOKY

Standing straight and tall, look over your right shoulder as far as you can without straining or discomfort, then look over your left shoulder as far as you can without discomfort. Continue alternating back and forth smoothly and easily between the two positions.

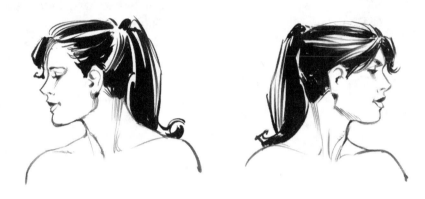

THE DOWN AND NEUTRAL

Standing straight and tall, gently tuck your chin into your chest and then straighten your head back up to neutral so that your eyes are gazing straight forward. Alternate back and forth between these two positions without straining the back of your neck.

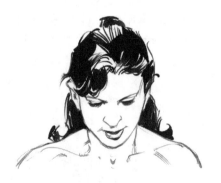
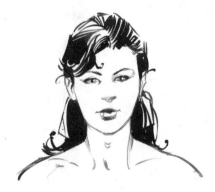

THE UP AND DOWN

Standing up straight and tall, raise your shoulders toward your ears and lower them back down. Repeat the movement several times, allowing your shoulders to relax down more and more each time.

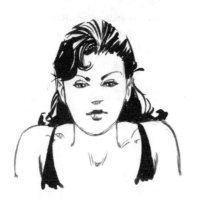 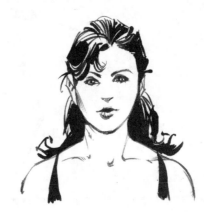

SHOULDER ROLLS

Standing up straight and tall, roll both shoulders up, back, and down in a circular movement. Continue rolling several times, then reverse directions and roll the shoulders forward. Try to make the movement more fluid each time.

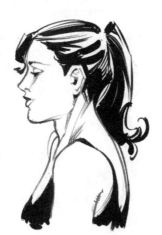 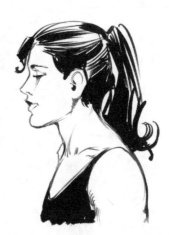

HAND CLAPS

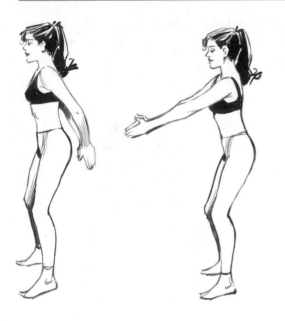

Standing straight and tall, keeping your elbows straight, swing your arms so that the hands come together clapping in front. Then swing them together so that they come as close as is comfortable in back. Alternate rhythmically between the two positions, allowing the shoulders to open up.

STANDING CAT STRETCHES

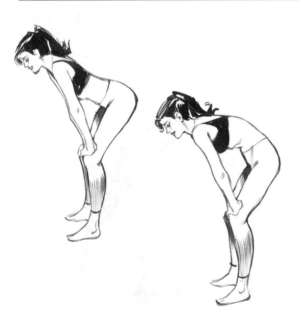

Bend forward from the hips, with the knees slightly bent. Keeping your hands on the tops of your thighs for support, round your back, drawing your belly button in toward your spine. As you exhale, round your back; as you inhale, lengthen your spine, tailbone, and neck. Alternate rhythmically between these two positions, allowing your spine to relax and lengthen.

TWIST AND REACH

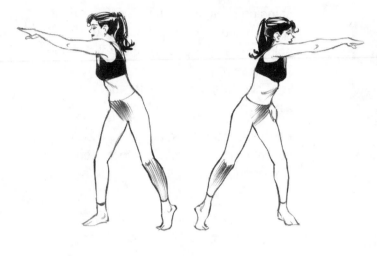

Stand with your feet hip-width apart and your arms down at your sides. Leaning your body weight into your left foot, reach to the left with your right arm, so that your right heel raises slightly off the floor. Then lean your body weight into your right foot, and reach to the right with your left arm, so that your left heel raises slightly off the floor. Alternate between both positions rhythmically, gradually making the movements bigger and more fluid.

TWIST AND REACH WITH ROTATION

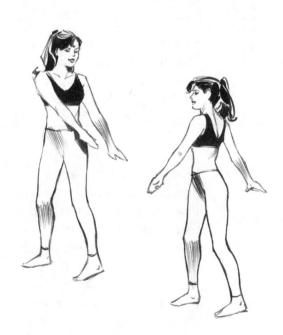

Perform the same movement that you did in the Twist and Reach; however, this time keep the arms alongside and slightly away from your body. Allow your waist to open and twist more as you warm up. Make the movements slowly and gently.

SIDE-TO-SIDE KNEE-UP WITH PULL-IN

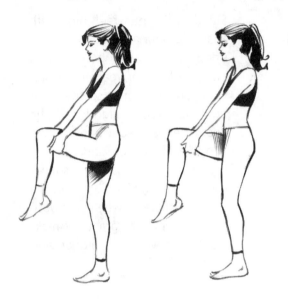

Standing straight and tall, raise your right knee up and draw it in toward your chest, holding it at the back of the right thigh. Then raise your left knee up and in toward your chest, holding it at the back of the left thigh.

Keep your spine as straight as possible as you alternate rhythmically between the two positions.

DANCING PONY BACK

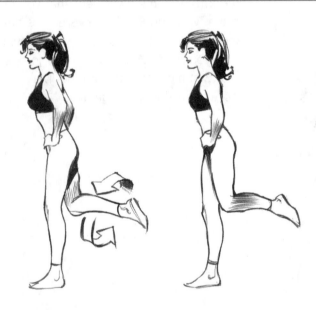

Standing straight and tall, bring your right heel up toward your buttocks and circle the right lower leg three times in a clockwise direction, moving from the hip. Lower your right leg and raise your left heel up toward your buttocks, circling the left heel three times in a counterclockwise direction. Change legs again, and this time rotate the right leg in a counterclockwise direction, then rotate the left leg in a clockwise direction. Continue to alternate between each of these positions, allowing the hips to release more and more each time.

GENTLE CAN-CANS

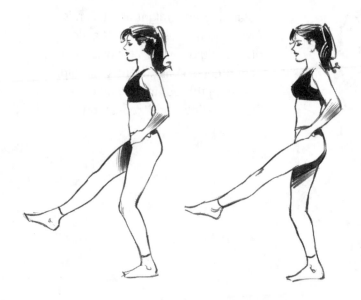

Stand straight and tall. Gently kick the legs out, alternating between the right and the left. These kicks should be performed slowly and easily, with the legs kept down low. Alternate back and forth between each of these two positions.

SLO-MO "KARATE KICKS"

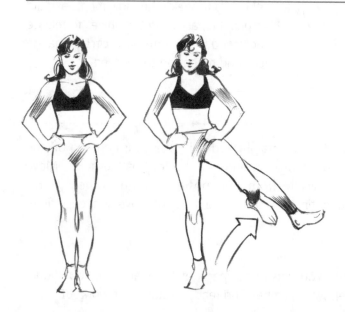

Standing on your left leg, lift your right leg directly out to the side with the knee bent, and with a controlled motion, straighten out the right knee in a slow motion "karate kick" move. Then transfer the weight onto your right leg, and repeat the movement with the left leg. Alternate rhythmically between the two positions.

PERFORMANCE TIP: Try not to lean over too much to the opposite side when you lift the leg. Try to keep your torso as upright as possible throughout the movements.

STANDING HIP CIRCLES

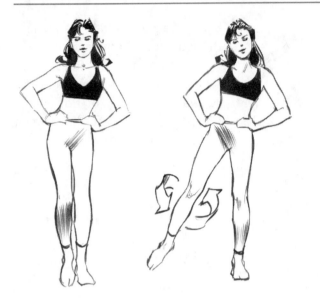

Standing up straight and tall, raise your right knee up off the floor. Make fluid circles clockwise and counterclockwise from your hip, keeping the leg up the entire time. Change legs and repeat on the opposite side.

ANKLE CIRCLES

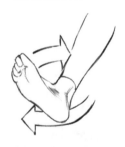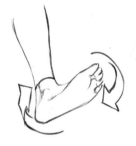

Standing up straight and tall, raise your right leg off the ground and circle the foot at the ankle in one direction, then in the other. Try to make the movements as fluid as possible, allowing the ankles to release more and more with each circle. Change legs and repeat on the left leg.

POINT AND FLEX

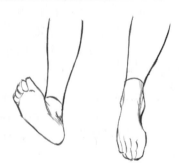

Standing up straight and tall, raise your right leg off the ground and point and flex the foot at the ankle. Move rhythmically from one position to the other, gently attempting to increase the range of movement each time.

● ● ●

Once you finish both parts of the warm-up, you should feel, warm, limber, and ready to start your workout.

Your Fit + Female Workout

At this point refer back to chapter 7 and the appropriate Fit + Female Workout for your body type (whether bare minimum, ideal, or gung-ho). After you finish your routine, come back to this chapter and we'll end with a relaxing cool-down.

The Cool-Down ●●●

The cool-down is typically the ugly stepchild of most exercise programs. People tend to put it to the side and forget about it. And that's perfectly understandable, because the last thing that anyone feels like doing at the end of the workout is more exercise. Nevertheless, the cool-down is a vital component of a safe and effective program.

The purpose of the cool-down (also called a "warm-down") is essentially the opposite of the warm-up, to gradually decrease the body temperature and the heart rate. The cool-down allows the body to gradually return to its normal resting state.

As with the warm-up, there are two basic parts to the cool-down. The first consists of gentle movements similar to what you were doing during the actual workout. The second part is a static stretch segment to improve flexibility and help remove waste products from the muscles. Let's take a look at each of the cool-down components in greater detail.

Step One: Easy Does It

After your workout (especially if you are doing intense cardiovascular exercise), it's extremely important to keep moving but at a dramatically reduced pace. If you were jogging, for example, your cool-down could be a slow walk. If you were cycling, your cool-down could be cycling, but at a slower pace. Whatever you choose, just be sure to keep your legs going for at least five minutes, while gradually decreasing your intensity. The most important thing is to not stop exercising suddenly.

The reason for this is that during cardiovascular exercise, there is a dramatic increase in blood flow to the muscles. Due to the structural nature of veins, whenever you stop moving abruptly, blood tends to pool in your legs and feet. This diverts blood from both your heart and your brain and can make you feel faint or dizzy. A properly structured cool-down allows the vascular system to recover from the workout more slowly, thereby reducing the chances of feeling unwell after exercise.

How can you tell if you're cooled down enough to stop moving? Well, one good guideline is to take your heart rate, and don't stop moving until the heart rate is below 120 beats per minute. For individuals who have never worked out before, it may take a great deal of time for the heart rate to return to normal, even 15 minutes or more. The good news is that as your fitness level improves, you will recover faster. This improvement can be seen in just a few weeks of regular activity.

Note: If your heart rate remains elevated for a prolonged period despite doing a moving cool-down, try sitting down or (if you feel unwell) lying down with your feet elevated until your heart rate is below 120 beats per minute. Also, if you ever feel ill (or unusually exhausted) after exercising, be sure to contact your physician immediately.

Step Two: Stretch and Lengthen

The second part of the cool-down is a flexibility segment that improves the ability of the muscles to lengthen and increases the range of motion possible around the joints. Immediately following a workout is an ideal time for this because muscles are warmer and therefore more pliable and responsive to stretch. Stretching has many benefits, including

Increasing the pliability of muscles and tendons

Increasing the range of motion in the joints

Reducing muscle tension

Developing body awareness

Promoting greater circulation

Decreasing stress

When performing each of the following stretches, simply get into position and hold it to the point of mild tension for 15 to 30 seconds. If the tension eases after that, slowly and gently move further into the stretch without straining until tension is felt again. Then hold it for another 15 seconds or more.

It's important to remember to breathe fully and deeply while stretching. When you start each stretch, try to exhale fully through your mouth. Once you feel the sensation of mild tension, hold the position and inhale deeply through the nose, then exhale through the mouth. Now we will go through each of the stretches in greater detail.

CALF STRETCH ON THE WALL

(stretches the calves)

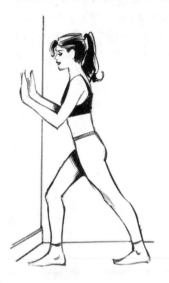

Standing with both hands against the wall, lunge forward with one leg, bending the front knee. Reach the back leg behind you and gently lower the heel to the floor, stretching the calf of the leg in back. Hold and breathe for 15 to 60 seconds. Repeat on the other side.

CHEST STRETCH ON THE DOOR

(stretches the chest and the front of the shoulders)

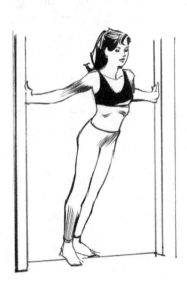

Stand with both feet inside of a doorway. Place both hands with the palms facing outward, thumbs up. Lean forward with your body weight stretching out your chest and the front of your shoulders. Breathe and hold for 15 to 60 seconds.

SIDE STRETCH STANDING

(stretches the back and the waist)

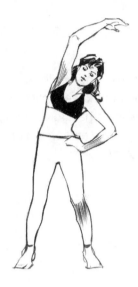

Stand with your feet wider than hip-width apart, place one hand on top of your hip, and raise the other arm over your head, reaching up and over to the other side. You should make a gentle arch with your body. Breathe deeply and hold for 15 to 60 seconds. Repeat on the other side.

CAT/COW

(stretches the back, the abdominals, the shoulders, and the hips)

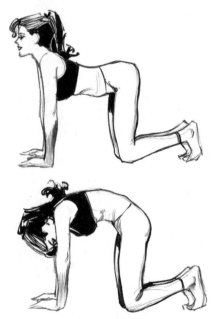

Kneel on all fours with your hands directly underneath your shoulders and your knees directly under your hips. Exhale and round your back, tucking your chin in toward your chest and your tailbone between your legs. Then inhale and lift your head, lengthening the back of your neck, allowing a gentle bend in your back, and lifting your tailbone. Gently alternate between the two positions several times, allowing your spine to limber and lengthen as you move.

SAFETY TIP: Don't arch your back too much. You should feel the stretch only in the muscles and have no discomfort whatsoever in the spine.

BUTTERFLY

(stretches the inner thighs)

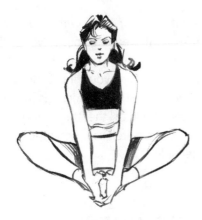

Sit up straight and tall on your sit bones with the soles of your feet touching. Gently allow your knees to fall out to the sides of the room, releasing the muscles of the inner thighs. Hold without bouncing for 15 to 60 seconds.

SIDE-LYING HIP FLEXOR/QUAD STRETCH

(stretches the top of the thigh and the hip)

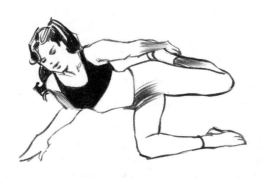

Lie on your side with your bottom thigh out in front of you at a 45-degree angle from your torso. Your bottom forearm and the palm of your hand should be down on the floor in front of you for support. Staying balanced on the hips, pull your abdominals in to protect your back, and use the top hand to gently draw the top heel in toward your buttocks. Try to line the top thigh up with your torso without straining.

PERFORMANCE TIP: Squeeze the buttocks together and press your pubic triangle forward to increase the stretch in the top of the thigh. Stay on your hip; if you absolutely have to lean, lean forward, not back.

LYING DOWN SINGLE KNEE TO CHEST

(stretches the buttocks, the lower back, and the back of the thigh)

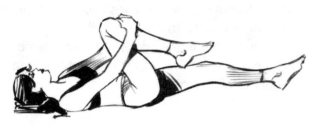

Lie flat on your back with your legs out straight. Keeping your lower back on the floor, bend your right knee and pull it in toward your chest. Breathe and hold for 30 to 60 seconds, allowing the back of the thigh and the lower back to release. Repeat on the other side.

LYING DOWN DOUBLE KNEES TO CHEST

(stretches the lower back)

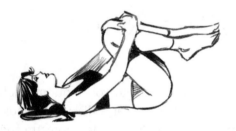

Lying on your back, draw both knees in toward your chest and release your lower back into the floor. Breathe and hold for 30 to 60 seconds.

MODIFIED MORNING STAR

(stretches the waist, the chest, and the outer thighs)

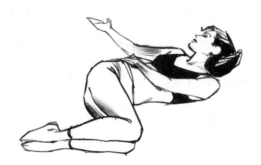

Begin by lying on your back. Bend your right knee and bring it in close to your chest, then cross it over your chest so that it makes a 45- to 90-degree angle with your torso. Place your left hand on your right hip to gently encourage your knee across the body. Breathe deeply and hold the stretch for 30 to 60 seconds. Repeat on the other side.

HAMSTRING STRETCH IN HOOK-LYING POSITION

(stretches the back of the thighs)

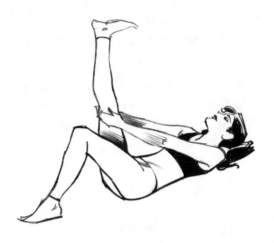

Lie on your back with both knees bent, your feet flat on the floor. Straighten your right leg and extend it toward the ceiling. Hold the back of the right leg with both hands and gently draw the leg in toward your chest until you feel a comfortable stretch on the back of the right leg. Breathe and relax into the stretch. Hold it for 30 to 60 seconds, then repeat this on the other side.

SAFETY TIP: Make sure that you feel the stretch in the back of the thigh and not behind the knee. If you feel the stretch behind the knee, bend it slightly and draw it in toward the chest.

PERFORMANCE TIP: If you have a difficult time holding onto the back of your thigh, wrap a rope or a belt around the arch of your foot and draw it in toward your chest.

FIGURE-FOUR STRETCH

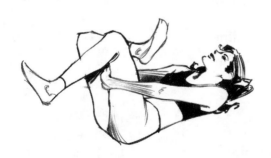

Lie on your back with both knees bent, your feet flat on the floor. Cross your right ankle, and rest it on top of your left thigh. Then take both hands and bring them together, holding the back of the thigh. Try to keep your hip rotated so that your right knee points out to the right side of the room. Breathe deeply and hold the stretch for 30 to 60 seconds. Repeat on the other side.

CORPSE POSE—BREATHE AND RELAX

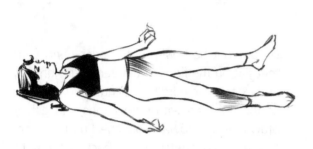

Lie on your back with your arms alongside your body and your palms facing upward. Your legs should be straight, hip-width apart. Allow your thighs to relax and your feet to gently fall open to the outsides of the room. Allow for the natural curvature in the lower body.

Relax and imagine that your body is sinking down into the floor. Breathe in deeply through your nose and out through your mouth.

Relax and Center

By the end of the cool-down, you will probably already feel calmer and more relaxed than you did before you started working out. This is because exercise actually activates the branch of your nervous system (known as the parasympathetic system) that regulates relaxation and calms down the bodily processes. Therefore, this is a perfect time to take a few moments for yourself just to clear your head, breathe, and relax.

For lack of a better word, this is actually a form of meditation at its most basic level, and it's surprisingly less complicated to do than people would believe. Here are just some of the benefits of taking a little relaxation downtime for yourself.

Reduced stress and anxiety

Reduced depression

Reduced irritability and moodiness

Feelings of vitality and rejuvenation

Increased emotional control

Increased self-esteem

Increased alertness

May help lower blood pressure

To try it, simply lie on your back in what is known as the corpse pose. Your arms should be at your sides, your legs straight but relaxed and opened naturally at the hips so that your feet turn out toward the sides of the room. There should be a natural curve in your neck and another in the small of your back. Now, just lie there and breathe, allowing your body to sink down into the floor. Try to think of nothing but the natural rhythm of the rise and fall of your own breath. Try to be in the moment, not thinking about the future, not thinking about the past. If you'd like, you can focus on a single word (or a mantra), such as *calm*, for example, saying it over and over in your mind as you breathe deeply and relax.

As thoughts drift in and out of your mind (and they certainly will), try to notice them without getting attached to them, just the way that you would notice clouds passing in the summer sky. Continue breathing and stay connected with your breath. That's all there is to it. That is the essence of meditation: relax, breathe, and be present.

The great thing about meditation (and stress-reduction techniques in general) is that a little goes a long way. If you can find even 5 or 10 minutes per day (and not necessarily at the end of your workout), you will reap incredible benefits in relaxation and stress reduction.

Not by Workouts Alone ●●●

Exercise is only half of the fitness equation—eating right is the other. Without a healthful and balanced approach to nutrition, even the most dedicated exerciser will inevitably be disappointed with her results.

The first step in changing your eating patterns is getting rid of any misconceptions you may have about what constitutes a proper diet. Many of us, regardless of our body types, have ideas about food and eating that range from untrue to ineffective to downright dangerous. Before we discuss specific food programs for each body type, let's first examine a few of these faulty beliefs and detail some new, more empowering options for developing a healthier relationship with food.

9

how to think about diets and dieting

Nearly everywhere you go, from locker rooms to office water coolers to the local Gymboree class, it seems that whenever women gather together, the conversation eventually turns to the subject of dieting. Someone may be talking about the diet that she is currently on, the diet she knows she should go on, or perhaps the diet that helped her friend lose twenty pounds in a month.

If you mention an effective diet plan, all the ears in the room will prick up as if they've heard a hot stock tip. Everyone wants to know about the latest and greatest diet plan. Human nature being what it is, we all want to believe that there is a newly uncovered mystery that reveals the secrets of quick and easy weight loss. As a society, we are always looking for that magic bullet, so much so that weight loss is currently a $50 billion industry. From Atkins to the Zone to the South Beach Diet to (my personal favorite) the Cabbage Soup Diet, there is no shortage of diets on the market, with new ones popping up almost every day.

Ironically, despite this obsession with diets, 60 percent of the U.S. population is currently overweight and diets have an overall failure rate of 95 percent! Why? Well, one main reason is that most diets don't teach you how to eat for the rest of your life. They simply offer you a plan, a quick fix that may or may not work in the short term. Unfortunately, the real challenge is not necessarily losing weight; it's being able to keep it off for the long haul.

When you talk to people who are successful at losing weight and keeping it off, they will almost always tell you that they have made some fundamental shifts, not only in terms of what they eat, but also in the way they think about food. Interestingly enough, whenever I counsel clients about their nutritional problems, several patterns come up time and time again. The fact is, many of us share the same self-defeating beliefs and behaviors that cause us to derail our weight-loss efforts. I call these the diet traps.

Rather than having my clients choose a particular diet, I always ask them to take stock of what their bad habits are and try to correct them. Instead of reinventing the wheel and trying to eat in a completely different way, it's easier and more realistic to analyze what you are currently doing and see what isn't working.

The key is to be willing to take a hard look at yourself and your motivations. Unfortunately, diet is one area where many of us are not really honest with ourselves about the things we do that undermine our ability to lose weight and keep it off. The only way that you can change whatever isn't working is to be honest about it.

Let's look at the diet traps in greater detail. As we go through the list, try to be as truthful as possible about which of these traps have snared you over the years.

The Diet Traps ●●●

Diet Trap #1: "I'm working out, so I can eat more."

The Belief: "I worked out today. I know I burned a ton of calories, so I should be able to indulge in this ——— (insert indulgence of choice—hot fudge sundae, bag of potato chips, margarita, etc.)."

The Reality: Exercise does help burn calories but not nearly as many as people would like to believe. Moreover, exercise alone is rarely a successful road to weight loss. It almost always takes some dietary restrictions, too. The average workout of cardio, resistance, and flexibility probably burns between 300 and 600 calories. Do that five days a week, and you are burning about a half a pound of fat from exercise.

However, because of the high calorie counts of many popular foods, it's surprisingly easy to undo the efforts of your exercise program with just a few poorly chosen mouthfuls. For example, a Starbuck's Mocha Frappuccino (which many women view as just another cup of joe) is approximately 300 calories. This means that with just a few quick sips, you could completely trash all of the calorie-burning benefits of your workout.

Of course, a treat here and there is a healthful and appropriate part of a balanced life, but unfortunately, unless you are an ultra-marathoner, working out is usually not a license to eat anything you want. Those of us who need to watch our weight (this includes endo-pears, endo-apples, and, to a lesser extent, meso-pears and meso-apples) must make smarter choices every day.

Diet Trap #2: "My husband is a 'meat and potatoes' man."

The Belief: "My husband won't eat any of that diet rabbit-food stuff. He's a real 'meat and potatoes' kind of guy. The problem is that when I cook the kind of food he likes to eat, I end up gaining weight."

The Reality: Your husband has the right to be any kind of man that he wants to be, but you also have the right and the power to make your own choices.

Certainly, "meat and potatoes" men aren't the most healthful eaters on the planet. By definition, these guys tend not to eat nearly enough fruits, vegetables, and whole grains. Many of them are overweight, and even those who aren't will probably have long-term health complications related (at least in part) to a poor diet. From high cholesterol to type 2 diabetes to cancers to GI issues to lack of overall energy, a poor diet can really take its toll on the human body.

So, if this is your husband's pattern, it's actually in his best interests to make some changes; however, you can't force him to do something he's not interested in. It's like that old saying, "You can lead the horse to the table, but you can't make him eat the tofu and carrot sticks." You can encourage, cajole, and even nag, but if it's something that he doesn't want to do for himself, it just won't happen.

That said, your husband's choices don't have to be your choices. As a wife and a mother, I completely understand the desire to take care of and do things for the people you love. However, there are ways to do your own thing while at the same time meeting the needs of the people you care about.

Let's say, for example, that his meal of choice is a big, greasy slab of red meat and French fries. Serve him (or, better yet, teach him how to cook for himself) whatever he wants but modify the meal for yourself. Choose a leaner cut of meat, watch your portion sizes (more about this later), have a baked sweet potato instead of fries, and throw in a big green salad or lots of veggies to go with it. It's up to you. You're an adult woman, well past the age where people can try to force-feed you. The bottom line is that you don't have to lose control of your diet because of someone else's choices.

Diet Trap #3: "I have no time for myself."

The Belief: "I would love to take better care of myself and eat right, but I'm so busy with my family (my job, the house, etc.) that I just don't have enough time to eat right, much less exercise."

The Reality: I have yet to meet the woman who has enough time for herself. I don't care who she is. Think about it, how many times in your life have you had just oodles of time with nothing to do? Not many, I'm guessing.

Speaking from personal experience, I don't know that I've ever felt like I had all the time in the world. In high school, I was trying to get good grades and get into a decent college, plus working part time. In college, I was trying to do well in school, plus working part time. As a woman entering the working world, I wanted to get ahead in my career (initially, advertising and public relations), and I put a good deal of effort into that. Then in graduate school, I was working and going to school full time. Now I'm married and a mom, and I work full time. You get the picture. There is always something going on in our lives. Time is limited and precious for everyone. The idea that we will ever have the world stop or slow down for us so that we can get it all together is an illusion. Let go of it.

We don't have the luxury of waiting around for the day when we will suddenly have a relaxed life with lots of time for ourselves. Chances are, over time, we're going to take on even more responsibility with our families, our careers, and so on. In the future, most of us should expect to have even less free time, not more.

The great irony is that if we don't take care of our bodies through sound nutrition and exercise, we won't have the health and the vitality to accomplish all of the things we want to do anyway.

Besides, at the risk of sounding shallow, part of feeling good about yourself is aesthetic, feeling good about the way you look. If you don't take care of yourself, you'll likely not only feel worse, but you'll look worse, too. This starts a vicious cycle of despair and self-loathing. Eventually, you'll stop believing that you have a right to take care of yourself at all.

There will probably never be a point in time where we can just put our lives on hold and pull things together. This means we need to commit to improving our eating patterns in our current situation. We need to find ways to eat right and exercise consistently in the environment that we find ourselves in right now. No matter how crazed your day-to-day situation may be, there is always a way to at least improve your dietary habits, if you're truly committed to making the effort. More about this in the next chapter.

Diet Trap #4: " I've tried to starve myself, but I can't."

The Belief: "I really want to lose weight. I know that if I could just stop eating for a few days, I would be able to drop a few pounds easily. Several times in the past, like when I've gotten sick with a stomach flu, for example, I've actually lost a few pounds in the process. Of course, I don't like being sick, but that initial weight loss of a few pounds seems to shrink my stomach and motivates me to stay on track to keep losing weight."

The Reality: Your body needs a certain number of calories just to keep running. The bare minimum of calories your body needs to survive in a resting state is called the resting metabolic rate. When you take in fewer calories than you need (as is the case with fasting, liquid diets, or very-low-calorie diets), your body actually goes into starvation mode and lowers your metabolic rate to ensure your survival.

Taking in too few calories is particularly taxing on the brain and the skeletal muscles. The brain and the muscles must have adequate blood sugar for normal functioning. If you don't get enough blood sugar from the breakdown of the foods you eat, your body will draw on its own storage form of carbohydrates, known as glycogen.

Glycogen is found in liver and muscle tissue. Because glycogen is stored with three to four times its weight in water, whenever your body breaks down a pound of glycogen, you will lose approximately three pounds of water weight with it. This is why so-called crash dieting is so popular—you lose a lot of water weight in a very short period of time. While this type of weight loss is certainly fast, it's also very unhealthful—and it doesn't last.

Excessive water loss from crash dieting can contribute to dehydration and the loss of electrolytes. Electrolytes are minerals that are essential for nerve transmission, muscle contraction, and the regulation of bodily fluids. Severe electrolyte imbalances can even be fatal.

Most important, as soon as you start to eat normally, all that water weight will (and ought to) be replaced. Starvation diets also lead to irritability, mental confusion, gastrointestinal problems, and the loss of lean body mass. As I mentioned earlier, the loss of each pound of lean body tissue means that you burn 30 to 50 less calories per day. So if you lose several pounds of lean body tissue from crash dieting, you could decrease your metabolism's ability to burn several hundred calories per day. Again, over time this can contribute to a substantial weight gain, making it much easier to pack on the pounds and harder to burn them off.

Of course, caloric restriction is a necessary part of weight loss. The reason that any diet ever works is ultimately the same: you take in fewer calories than you expend. Period. None the less, you need to eat at least the bare minimum of calories to allow your body to function, or you risk doing damage to your metabolism and your health.

Diet Trap #5: "Eating is one of my few pleasures".

The Belief: "I work really hard, I have very little time to myself, and eating is one of the few things in life that I enjoy. I really look forward to having a glass or two of wine, a delicious meal, and a wonderful dessert. I feel like I deserve it. For all that I do for everyone else, this is a way of doing something nice just for me. I'm not going to give that up."

The Reality: No one will argue that food isn't one of life's greatest pleasures, but that is not food's primary role. Ultimately, food is fuel for your body. Your body needs the proper nutrients to function and maintain health. Many of the meals that we treat ourselves with actually do harm to our bodies, in both the short and the long term.

Take, for example, the kind of meal that people eat when they want to indulge themselves. Let's say the meal consists of

A fried calamari appetizer

Two buttered rolls

An entrée of fettuccini Alfredo

Tiramisu for dessert

Two glasses of red wine

While there is no doubt that this meal will taste delicious, nutritionally speaking it is a total nightmare!

First of all, it doesn't provide much in the way of immediate nutrition. The meal is loaded with fat and contains no fresh fruits or vegetables, no fiber, tons of processed white flour, and a boatload of empty calories. The energy total for this meal is a staggering 2,600 calories.

Keep in mind that the average woman needs about 2,000 to 2,100 calories per day, and this one meal alone provides 500 to 600 calories more than that! In this meal, 63 percent of the calories are from fat and almost all of it is heart-hostile saturated fat.

Toss in a 400-calorie breakfast and a 700-calorie lunch, and you're looking at 3,700 calories for the day—or about 1,600 calories more than is probably required. That's equal to a half-pound weight gain from just one bad day alone! It's easy to see how a few of those days strung together could result in a substantial weight gain in no time.

The bottom line is that this meal is a treat for your tastebuds but an assault on your body. Eat too many meals like it too often, and over time (unless you are genetically blessed), you will most likely (at the very least) develop high blood cholesterol, significant weight gain, and eventually, perhaps high blood pressure and cardiovascular disease.

If you would like to do something good for yourself, consider some other options: schedule a massage, get a manicure and a pedicure, buy yourself a new outfit or a pair of shoes, take a nice long bubble bath, or curl up with a trashy novel. All of these are indulgences that feed your soul without filling up your fat cells and clogging your arteries.

Diet Trap #6: "There's no 'real food' in my diet."

The Belief: "I can only eat the stuff that I'm in the mood to eat, things that taste good. I know all the things that I should be eating, but I never do. I've always been like this. I'm such a junk-food junkie, my friends are always goofing on me."

The Reality: This is similar to the "Eating Is One of My Few Pleasures" Trap, but instead of making a poor choice of food a few times a week or even once a day, women who fall into this trap basically eat garbage all day long.

For some women, it's high-calorie junk; for others it's low-calorie junk, but basically with this trap there are no nutrient-rich foods in the diet at all.

I can relate to this scenario in particular because I used to eat this way. At one point in my life, I was interested only in whether the food tasted good; I didn't care in the least whether it was good for me or whether it nourished my body. I never viewed food as the fuel that it is. Here is a typical diet for another woman I know who still eats like this on a daily basis:

Breakfast: A diet iced tea and a doughnut

Snack: A blueberry muffin with butter and a cup of coffee

Lunch: Some French fries and a chocolate milkshake

Snack: A Snickers bar

Dinner: A slice of pizza and a diet Coke

This diet contains about 2,400 calories of basically zero nutrients. It consists of highly processed sugar, no green veggies, no orange or yellow veggies, not enough protein, virtually no fiber, and virtually no fruit, almost half of its calories are from fat (most of it saturated), it has not nearly enough water, and it has lots and lots of chemicals. And yet many women eat like this every day. A diet like this would result in low energy levels and dips in energy levels throughout the day and nutritional deficiencies over time.

Diet Trap #7: "Once I start eating that, I can't stop."

The Belief: "There are some foods that I just can't control myself with—like ice cream, for example. I can't ever seem to eat just one scoop. I start out with one scoop, but I keep eating more and more. Before I know it, I've finished the entire container. It's so bad that I continue eating even after I feel over-full and a bit sick."

The Reality: For many of us, there are certain trigger foods that we just can't seem to control ourselves around. One bite leads to another and another until we literally feel that we can't stop eating.

Generally speaking, the trigger foods tend to be so-called comfort foods and are typically high in fat, sugar, or both. Whether the food is chocolate, potato chips, candy, popcorn, cookies, or nuts, most of us have at least one food that once we start eating it, we can't seem to stop. This problem of trigger foods is particularly complicated because it appears that there are both psychological and physiological reasons for these cravings.

On the psychological side, this binge eating is often a way to deal with painful or uncomfortable emotions, such as stress, anger, anxiety, sadness, loneliness, and even boredom. A lot of this is a learned response from our earliest childhoods. Babies are given mother's milk or bottles to pacify them. Kids are given sweets as a reward for good behavior or to cheer them up when they feel down. Foods that taste good provide a temporary pleasant experience that offers an enjoyable diversion from life's troubles. Unfortunately, when these feel-good foods are eaten to excess, this short-lived feeling of calmness is often followed by feelings of deep regret and self-loathing because one has overeaten.

In addition, there is evidence that real physiological reasons exist for overindulging in comfort foods. Some of these foods actually contain chemicals that alter brain chemistry. Chocolate, for example, contains more than 300 different constituent compounds, including anandamide, which has effects on the brain that are similar to those of marijuana and hashish.

Carbohydrates can improve one's mood by increasing the levels of the neurotransmitter (brain chemical) serotonin. High levels of serotonin in the brain are associated with relaxation, satisfaction, and feelings of happiness and well-being. Low levels of serotonin are associated with depression. Experts believe that individuals with low serotonin levels may have sugar cravings as their bodies try to regulate their neurochemistry and improve their mood. In fact, serotonin levels drop just before a woman gets her period, and they have been implicated as a factor in the mood swings of premenstrual syndrome (PMS). The overeating (especially of high-carb foods) that many women indulge in just before their periods begin may be an attempt by the body to reduce these feelings of depression. Many antidepressant medications are designed to do the same thing: increase serotonin levels in the brain and thereby improve mood.

We also know that carbohydrates are responsible for elevating blood sugar levels. Having low blood sugar alone is associated with irritability and fatigue.

Although many women succumb to the occasional pig-out (which may cause frustration and may derail weight-loss efforts), overeating can also be a sign of several psychological disorders, including bulimia nervosa and binge-eating disorder. Signs of a binge-eating disorder include

Eating large amounts of food when you are not hungry

Overeating to the point of being uncomfortably full

Eating beyond what most people would eat in a given amount of time and/or under similar circumstances

Engaging in these behaviors at least two times per week for six months or more

Regular use of compensatory behaviors in an attempt to counteract the effect of overeating, such as vomiting, the use of laxatives or diuretics, excessive exercise, or fasting

Eating food very rapidly

Eating alone because of embarrassment about how much you are eating

If you or someone you care about engages in any of these behaviors, please seek medical attention immediately. There are many treatments available for eating disorders. Get professional help from your doctor as soon as possible, to avoid potentially life-threatening health problems.

If overeating is not indicative of a more serious health problem, there are several things you can do to avoid pigging out on trigger foods:

Learn to enjoy a small amount of the food when you feel the craving. Portion control it, savor the taste, and enjoy it slowly.

Find substitutions for the craving—for example, low-fat microwave Kettle Corn (sweet popcorn, similar to Cracker Jacks), chocolate- or caramel-flavored rice cakes, diet hot cocoa, or a few mini-sized candy bars

Try waiting fifteen minutes before giving in to a craving by distracting yourself with another activity, such as writing in a journal, exercising, listening to music, or taking a little catnap. Sometimes even five minutes of distraction is enough to prevent you from overdoing it.

If, however, like most of us, you occasionally give in to a craving and eat more than you want to, don't beat yourself up. We are all human, and it's perfectly normal to get a little out of control every once and a while. Rather than wallow in self-hatred or disgust, try to create an empowering strategy for yourself to prevent the behavior the next time. Ask yourself

Why did I do this? What set me off in the first place? Was I depressed, anxious, tired, or frustrated?

What else could I have chosen to do instead? Try to think of all the empowering behaviors you could have substituted for the pig-out that would make you feel better immediately instead of bad or guilty later on. List as many as possible, so that you have an arsenal at your disposal the next time you feel out of control with food.

All that said, occasionally you may just want to go a little bit overboard. And you know what? That's perfectly fine. We are human; sometimes it's fun to go a bit crazy. Just make sure it's not an everyday thing.

More important, if you do choose to overeat a bit, do so consciously. In other words, make a choice to do it so that you are in control of your behavior.

I actually do this every once in a while (especially if it's that time of the month), and I usually do it with chocolate. I make a conscious decision to go totally off the rails.

At times like this, here's an example of my internal dialogue: "I'm going to eat this entire bag of peanut M&Ms. I know that it's way too many calories and that it's not a healthful choice, but I'm giving myself permission to do this right now. For whatever reasons, this is what I feel that I need for myself at this moment. I'm going to do it, I'm going to enjoy it, I'm not going to feel guilty about it afterward, and I'm going to move on when I'm done."

Truly, if this is a once-in-a-blue-moon activity, it won't cause any short- or long-term damage to your health, your diet, your waistline, or your psyche. Again, though, the key is to do it because you choose to. You should be in control of the behavior; the behavior should not be in control of you.

Being in control of your food choices is the secret to lifelong healthful eating and easy weight maintenance. Talk to someone who has lost weight and successfully kept it off (in a healthful way), and you'll hear some common themes time and time again. These women will usually tell you that they feel very much in control of their food choices. No matter where these women are and no matter what choices are available to them at any given time, they are able to pick the best options. I call these choices "eating strategies."

Being in Control ●●●

Eating strategies are a series of plans that help you maintain an appropriate body weight without a lot of stress. They help you make consistent decisions on a daily basis that support your health and allow you to manage your weight. Eating strategies are fundamentally different from diets in several ways.

For one thing, being on a diet means that you are following someone else's prescribed plan. When you diet, the diet provides the rules and the regulations, and you are expected to follow them without questioning whether they make sense. These rules can include anything from "three bowls of cabbage soup per day" (mmmm . . . yummy) to "absolutely no carbohydrates for two weeks." Yet most of these directives are just a gimmick to sell a book, a program, and/or a brand of food products. These rules are just a way for someone else to make money off your desire to lose weight by hooking you into following his or her "magic formula."

There is nothing magical and mysterious about weight loss. Ultimately, all diets work for exactly the same reason. Weight loss happens because your body burns more calories than you take in, plain and simple. It could be because you eat only a few bowls of soup per day or because your portion sizes are dramatically smaller than normal, but at the end of the day, pounds are shed because you ate fewer calories than you did before and/or because you burned off more calories with exercise.

Once you take the hocus-pocus factor out of dieting, you can focus instead on understanding established nutritional truths and principles. As in other areas, when it comes to eating right, knowledge truly is power. Once you know what things work and why, you become the expert. Now you are in control. Rather than relying on someone else's solutions, you are now your own diet guru, and you are empowered to make the best choices for yourself every single day.

It often reminds me of that scene in *The Wizard of Oz*, when Dorothy, the Cowardly Lion, the Scarecrow, and the Tin Woodsman all see "the Great and Powerful Oz" for the first time. He is a scary giant green face on a screen, and they are all very frightened and awed. They soon learn however, that he is just a little, unassuming man pushing buttons from behind a curtain. There is nothing mysterious about him in the least, nothing to be nervous about. The same is true with weight loss; once you learn the eating strategies to control and maintain your weight, you won't ever be intimidated by the process again.

The Eating Strategies

Eating Strategy #1: Eat consciously.

Whenever you eat, be aware that you are eating. Whether it's a meal or a snack, mindless eating can wreak havoc with your diet. Examples of mindless eating include eating while standing up in the kitchen, munching at your desk or while driving, snacking in front of the TV or at the movies, and eating food off your kids' or spouse's plate.

Try instead to make eating a conscious process. Every time you eat, whether it's a meal or a snack, make sure that you are fully present in the moment. As women, most of the time we are multitasking, eating and doing something else at the same time. When we eat like that, it's easy to consume hundreds of calories and hardly be aware that we're doing it. For body types like meso-apples and meso-pears, who typically don't have too much of a struggle with weight, these several hundred calories might be the difference between maintaining weight and gaining weight.

What to Do
Eliminate all distractions. When you eat, make that the primary activity, not the secondary (or even tertiary) activity. Sit down, turn off the television, put down the book, get off the phone, stop the car, and focus completely on your meal.

Practice eating meditation. This is actually a practice from the ancient Buddhist meditative traditions. Like regular meditation, it involves being fully present in the moment, but rather than focusing on breathing, you focus on the act of eating. Because you want as few distractions as possible, this meditation works best when you dine alone. In order to practice eating meditation, try these simple steps:

Take a deep breath and release it, slowly.

Begin eating your meal.

With each mouthful, be aware of how you chew your food.

Think about how the food tastes.

Fully experience and enjoy every mouthful.

Don't rush.

Try to do this at least once a day for two weeks (even if it's just for a snack). Most likely, you'll develop a different approach to eating. Many people find that they automatically eat less when they eat this way, because they are aware of the sensation of being satisfied, and they stop eating before they are overfull.

Eating Strategy #2: Be honest with yourself.

One of the biggest problems that women have with controlling their weight is that they aren't completely honest with themselves about how much they eat. Some women deliberately delude themselves about how much they're eating, and others are truly clueless about the number of calories in the foods they eat. Either way, most people dramatically underestimate how much they eat. In fact, research suggests that most of us underestimate how much we eat by at least 20 percent!

In one interesting study, a researcher analyzed the diets of people who had been dieting but who reported difficulty in losing weight. Most of the dieters in the study said that they ate only 1,000 calories a day. When the experts monitored their food intake, however, the results showed that they actually ate two to three times that amount. In other words, they consumed 2,000 to 3,000 calories a day. It's no wonder they had difficulty losing weight!

What to Do

Keep a food and exercise journal. Studies suggest that people who keep a written record of what they eat (1) lose more weight, and (2) are more successful at keeping it off than those who don't. Food journals make you accountable for what you actually eat and make you aware of patterns that you might not notice otherwise.

For one full week (preferably two), keep a food log, a written record of everything you eat in the course of the day. The journal should include

1. What you ate (including the breakdown of combination foods like tunafish salad: 3 oz. of tuna, 2 tbs. of mayo, $\frac{1}{2}$ cup of veggies, etc.).

2. How much you ate. (What were the portion sizes? More on estimating portion sizes later.)

3. What time you ate it.

4. Where you were when you ate it.

5. Who you were with while you were eating.

6. How you felt at the time.

7. What you drank (water, soda, alcohol) and how much.

8. Any vitamins or supplements you consumed.

9. Any exercise you did during the day.

What's important is to be as thorough and honest as possible. If you're not, you are only cheating yourself. Remember, every single thing that you put into your mouth counts.

Here's an example of a breakfast entry in my client Sue's food log:

Breakfast: Monday, July 7th, 7 A.M.

(at home, with family, felt tired/sleepy)

2 cups of oatmeal

$\frac{1}{2}$ cup 1% milk

2 teaspoons of sugar

1 piece whole wheat toast

2 tablespoons of peanut butter

$\frac{1}{2}$ cup of blueberries

1 cup coffee w/2 tablespoons of milk and Equal

After you finish your journal, take some time to review your patterns. This can be done every day or every few days. See what you are doing that's working and what you might be able to improve upon. Here are a few things to consider when you look over your log.

Did you eat breakfast? We've all heard that breakfast is the most important meal of the day, and it's true. A recent study published in the *American Journal of Epidemiology* found that individuals who skipped breakfast were 4.5 times more likely to be obese than were people who regularly ate breakfast. Also, daily calorie intake was higher on days when people skipped breakfast.

Did you go more than five hours without eating? The same study that found breakfast skippers were more likely to be obese also found that in general, people who ate more frequent meals were thinner. In fact, those who had four or more meals per day were 45 percent less likely to be obese than were individuals who reported eating three or less.

Going too long between meals isn't a good idea for several reasons. For one thing, the act of digesting our food is actually responsible for about 10 percent of our metabolic rate. Eating small meals throughout the day takes advantage of this and keeps our metabolism chugging along all day. For another, when we go too long without eating, we tend to get over-hungry. Then, when we are ravenous, we are more likely to eat higher-calorie foods and to overeat. A good rule of thumb is to try for five small meals per day: breakfast, mid-morning snack, lunch, mid-afternoon snack, and dinner.

Did you get five servings of fruits and vegetables each day? Ideally, this breaks down to three servings of vegetables and two of fruit. The less that your fruits and veggies have been processed, the better. Try for raw, steamed, broiled, baked, or stir-fried. Stay away from deep-fried vegetables and fatty toppings such as cheese, oils, or butter.

Did you get at least six servings of whole grains each day? Whole grains are complex carbohydrates that benefit your body in two major ways. First, they serve as the primary energy source for the body by providing a steady release of energy. Second, because whole grains are in their whole form, they contain fiber, which has been shown to reduce the risks of developing heart disease, stroke, cancer, diabetes, and obesity. Whole grains include foods like wheat, corn, rice, oats, barley, quinoa, sorghum, spelt, rye, and even popcorn! Avoid heavily processed complex carbohydrates. The outer layer of the whole grain is removed in white flour products, taking with it protein and at least seventeen vitamins and minerals.

Did you get two to three servings of low-fat or fat-free dairy products each day? These include low-fat and fat-free milk, cheese, and yogurt. Dairy is important for bone health (such as for the prevention of osteoporosis) and has been linked to reducing the risk of hypertension, colon cancer, and obesity.

How much fat did you eat? And what kind? Experts recommend that no more than 30 percent of your daily calories should come from fat. The American Heart Association suggests that most of this fat, or about 15 percent of your total daily calories, should come from heart-healthy monounsaturated fats. Monounsaturated fats are found in olive, canola, and peanut oils, as well as in avocados. About 10 percent should come from polyunsaturated fats. Polyunsaturated fats include safflower, corn, and soybean oil, and soft margarine. No more than 10 percent should come from saturated fat. Saturated fats are usually (but not always) from animal sources and include lard, butter, whole-dairy products, and palm and coconut oils.

How much water did you drink? Between 60 and 70 percent of the human body is made up of water. The fact that we can survive for almost two months without food but only a few days without water underscores the importance of proper hydration. Water is essential for most bodily functions, including metabolism. It has been estimated that even mild dehydration can slow down the metabolic process by as much as 3 percent. If that doesn't sound like a lot, consider that the average woman requires about 2,000 calories per day. Three percent of that is 60 calories. Although 60 calories a day doesn't seem like much, at the end of one month it could result in a half pound of weight gain from dehydration alone—or about 6 pounds of weight gain in a year!

The challenge with dehydration is that the thirst sensation in most people is so weak, it's often confused with hunger. Many times we eat when what we really need to do is drink—water, that is. In a University of Washington study, an 8-ounce glass of water ended midnight "hunger pains" for 100 percent of the subjects.

That's why it's important to drink eight to ten 8-ounce glasses of water per day. One easy way to do this is to have a glass with each of your five to six small meals. By doing that, not only will you be more than halfway toward getting your eight glasses, you will probably find that you eat a good deal less than you normally would.

Eating Strategy #3: Don't be a member of the "Clean Plate Club."

When I was a little kid, I had a plate (with an angel's face on it) that said, "Be an Angel, Eat It All." My parents told me that I should finish all of my food because children were starving in Biafra. Now, I wasn't exactly sure where Biafra was (it sounded very far away), but it made me very sad to think that kids were starving over there. Moreover, I wasn't exactly sure how my finishing the creamed spinach would help them out. If anything, I used to try to think of how I might ship my creamed spinach to them so that they wouldn't be hungry anymore.

I think that as adults, many of us still subconsciously follow this line of fuzzy logic. Obviously, as an adult you realize that finishing all of the food on your plate won't affect anyone's situation but yours. Certainly, nobody wants to waste food; however, you also don't need to be a human garbage disposal, eating all the food on your plate or on someone else's.

In this country, portion sizes are considerably larger than they are in other countries. A New York University study found that the size of packaged foods and typical restaurant serving sizes exceeded standard portions by as much as eight times.

Researchers have recently become interested in "the French Paradox." Why do heart disease and obesity occur far less often in France than in this country, despite the French diet being relatively high in saturated fat? To examine whether this was due to portion sizes, the journal *Psychological Sciences* did an analysis of the difference between portion sizes in Philadelphia and Paris, comparing supermarket items, home cooking, and restaurant fare. Interestingly, researchers found that the restaurant portion sizes in Philadelphia were 25 percent bigger, on average. In fact, the Philadelphia serving sizes were larger in all cases but one; the French actually ate larger portions of vegetables. Another fascinating finding was that Parisians spend an average of 22 minutes consuming a meal, whereas Philadelphians spend an average of 14 minutes. By eating more slowly, the French make a smaller quantity of food last longer.

Larger servings actually entice people to eat more, even when they are no longer hungry. In a study published in *Obesity Research*, people didn't notice that they were served a portion size that was 50 percent larger than one they had been served (on the same plate) on the previous day. They ate 43 percent more calories with the larger serving size but made no mention of the size difference when questioned by researchers.

What to Do

So, how can you win the battle of the bulge when it seems that every-where you go, the supersizing of the American diet undermines your efforts? Here are some suggestions:

Order an appetizer as your entrée.

Share your entrée with someone.

When you place your order, tell your server that you'd like half of your entrée wrapped in a "to go" bag.

Don't buy the larger size of anything simply because it seems like a better deal. Remember that a good deal for your wallet may not be such a good deal for your waistline.

Eating Strategy #4: Combine the "Big Three."

There are three major classes of nutrients in the foods we eat: carbohy-drates, fats, and proteins. I call these the "Big Three."

Carbohydrates may be simple sugars (found in candy, sugar, fruits, and fruit juices) or complex carbohydrates (found in whole-grain products, vegetables, legumes, beans, and seeds). Their primary function in the body is to provide both short- and long-term energy. Most of our choices from this group should come from complex carbohydrates.

Fats are found in animal and plant sources, from vegetable oil to whole-milk cheese and meats. Animal fats are saturated fats, whereas fat from plants is usually polyunsaturated or monounsaturated.

Saturated fats are the most heart-hostile of all fats because they are associated with the buildup of plaque (a cholesterol-laden substance) that clogs arteries, leading to heart disease and stroke. Polyunsaturated fats are considered less unhealthful, but may be associated with an increased risk of cancer. Monounsaturated fats seem to be the most healthful fats of all. They can actually lower cholesterol levels and may protect against certain types of cancer.

Keep in mind that dietary fat is not a great evil. Fats are needed by the body to aid in the storage and the circulation of fat-soluble vitamins, promote healthy skin and hair, provide insulation for the body, and protect the vital organs. Our choices from the fat group need to be smart ones, however, which means that very little of the fat in our diets should come from saturated fat sources.

Protein, the last of the Big Three, is found in both animal and plant sources. Proteins are made up of building blocks called amino acids. There are twenty amino acids required by the human body. The body is able to make eleven of them on its own; however, nine of them cannot be produced internally and must be taken in through the diet. These are known as essential amino acids.

There are two types of protein: complete and incomplete. Animal protein is a complete protein, meaning that it contains sufficient amounts of all the essential amino acids to provide adequate nutrition. Vegetable proteins, on the other hand, are called incomplete proteins because they are missing one or more of the essential amino acids. If a wide variety of vegetable proteins are consumed however (as in the case of a healthful vegetarian diet), the body will get all of the essential amino acids that it needs. Protein is vital for tissue growth and maintenance, as well as for the production of antibodies, enzymes, and hormones.

What to Do

Ideally, you should try to eat a food from each of the Big Three at every meal. Eating a combination of protein, carbohydrates, and fats not only keeps blood sugar levels normal, it also provides a sustained release of energy. Carbohydrates help to supply immediate energy needs, and protein and fats provide longer-term energy. Also, because fats and protein are digested more slowly than carbohydrates, by adding a little of each to every meal you'll feel fuller, longer. Here are some examples of meals and snacks that contain foods from the Big Three:

> An egg white omelet with vegetables, whole wheat toast with soft margarine
>
> Whole-grain cereal with low-fat milk and blueberries
>
> Stir-fried chicken with vegetables and brown rice
>
> Salmon, salad with balsamic vinaigrette, and a baked sweet potato
>
> Whole-wheat crackers with peanut butter and a glass of skim milk

Eating Strategy #5: Eat as close to nature as possible.

One easy way of knowing that you are on the right track with your food choices is to eat as close to nature as possible. More often than not, if you choose food that is close to the way Mother Nature intended it, you won't go too far wrong. Why is that? Well, for one thing, foods in their natural state (by definition) have not been processed. Ironically, when we process foods, we tend to take out things that are good for us (like fiber, vitamins, and minerals) and put in things that are less good for us (such as sugar, saturated and polyunsaturated fats, and chemicals).

Not only are highly processed foods usually less nutritious, they contain additives. In most cases we don't know the long-term potential health risks associated with these chemicals. From saccharine to polyunsaturated fats, it seems like the list of substances added to our foods that may harm us over time just gets longer and longer.

One other benefit of foods in their raw state is that they have more phytochemicals. Phytochemicals (literally, "plant chemicals") are the substances in plants that prevent them from developing diseases. Interestingly enough, research suggests that these compounds may do the exact same thing for human beings. Plant foods in their most natural state will have more phytochemicals than those that are highly processed. More than nine hundred different phytochemicals have been identified so far. A single serving of vegetables may contain more than a hundred different phytochemicals!

Eating close to nature also means minimal cooking and food preparation and using as few added toppings as possible. This means steaming fish instead of deep-frying it in batter or having steamed veggies rather than veggies in a casserole with lots of added sauces.

Note: Obviously, some foods, such as poultry, beef, and shellfish, should always be well-cooked before being consumed to avoid the risk of food-borne illnesses.

What to Do
Look for the "naked food." Learn to identify the food with the least amount of processing and choose it, most of the time. Here are some examples:

Best Choice	Less Good Choice	Poor Choice
Fat-free cheese	Low-fat cheese	Whole-milk cheese
Apple	Applesauce	Apple turnovers
Baked potato (with skin)	Peeled, roasted potatoes	French fries
Water	Fruit juice	Soda
Steamed, baked, or stir-fried chicken	Steamed, baked or stir-fried chicken with sauce	Fried chicken

Ask yourself, "Is this addition to my food really necessary?" A good rule of thumb is, if you think you can live without adding it to your food, don't add it! Do you really need to add butter? If the answer is yes, do you really need to add that much? Or is there something more healthful, such as olive oil, that you could add instead? Whenever possible, try to pare down your food choice to its most basic state.

Eating Strategy #6: Move as much as possible.

Although this strategy doesn't have to do with food, it's crucial in terms of overall weight maintenance. We all know how important it is to be physically active; however, according to the U.S. Department of Health and Human Services, most adults and many children don't get enough regular physical exercise to provide them with any health benefits. This is defined as at least twenty minutes of moderate physical activity three times per week. Studies show that the more physically active an individual is, the lower his or her risk of premature death. This holds true for older as well as younger individuals.

Even if you can't exercise, you will derive benefits just from being physically active. Not only does increased physical activity reduce your chance of developing a chronic disease, it also burns more calories, which will help you maintain your weight. Keep in mind that about 70 percent of the calories we use every day are burned in the activities of daily living, or the ADLs. The more vigorous the ADLs are, the more calories you'll burn, and the easier it will be to lose weight and keep it off.

What to Do

Choose the more active choice whenever you can. This means walking as much as possible: in your house, when you have to run an errand, at the office, or across the parking lot. It means taking the stairs at the mall instead of the escalator or the elevator. It means turning your house cleaning into a "Let's see how much of my body I can get moving while I do this" activity. The more you move, the more calories you burn; the more calories you burn, the easier it is to stay trim.

Eating Strategy #7: Indulge yourself once in a while.

On the face of it, this strategy seems to contradict some of the others. Rather than telling you to stay on the straight and narrow all the time, I suggest that you let yourself go every once in a while.

Sometimes when you're being health-conscious, it's difficult to watch other people making choices that you wish you could make. For example, you're sitting at the restaurant eating your healthful meal of baked chicken and steamed veggies, while your dining companion is having a rich and delicious-looking plate of pasta in a creamy sauce that you figure has to pack at least 1,000 calories. Then you wonder why you can't do that. The truth is—you can! You have the right to do whatever you want to do. Just keep in mind that there are always consequences to every choice.

If you have made a lifestyle choice to feel and look a certain way, you can't make poor food choices on a daily basis. Even if you are an ecto-pear or an ecto-apple with a blast furnace for a metabolism and weight gain isn't an issue, poor food choices will ultimately have a negative effect on your health and vitality. You can't continually put the lowest quality "gasoline" into your "Ferrari" if you want to maintain a high-performance machine.

That said, it's a good idea to do something "bad" every once in a while, just because you choose to. It reminds you that you don't *have* to do anything. You can get as out of shape as you want and eat whatever you feel like eating, just as long as you are prepared to live with the consequences. Making a bad choice (whether it's pigging out on Grandma's three-cheese lasagna or Aunt Bessie's fried chicken or just deciding to blow off your workout that day) is actually a good thing to do every once in a while. You are reminded that you are the boss. Try to enjoy being bad while you're doing it, and when you're through (which, hopefully, is sooner rather than later), go back to being on track. If you're consistent with your program 80 to 90 percent of the time, you'll be successful. Doing anything 100 percent of the time quickly becomes stale and routine. A meditation teacher of mine was once asked whether it was okay to scratch yourself if you got an itch during meditation. "Absolutely," she said, "but scratch with a merry heart." In other words, make a choice to do it, go for it wholeheartedly, be fully present while you do it—and then get back to the business at hand at soon as possible.

In the next chapter, we'll build on these ideas as we look at specific eating guidelines for each body type.

how to eat for your body type: your body type eating plan

Despite what the Declaration of Independence says, all men (and women) are not created equal. Some of us just have an easier road to travel in many areas of our life—and weight control is one of them.

How many of us have watched our ecto-pear or ecto-apple sisters eat enough food to choke a horse and yet remain slim as gazelles? It doesn't seem fair. And you know what? It isn't. That's the way the proverbial cookie crumbles. Some people just have a faster metabolism and lots more leeway before they gain weight.

Take heart if you're not one of those people (and I'm certainly not), because you aren't alone. About 60 percent of the U.S. population is considered overweight. From a strictly Darwinian perspective, it's easy to see why we would be genetically programmed to hold on to body fat. More body fat means more storage energy in times of famine. Being able to withstand times of food scarcity ensures the survival of the species.

Having excess body fat is a problem, however, in terms of both health and esthetics. If you are not an ecto-apple or an ecto-pear, blessed with a mach 10 metabolism, fear not. There are many ways to lose weight and keep from putting it back on.

The previous chapter detailed eating strategies that work generally for most body types. Now let's examine more specific plans for each body type.

The Endo Plan ●●●

Both endo-pears and endo-apples have to be concerned with what health professionals call energy balance. Specifically, if they are trying to lose weight, they need to be in what is known as negative energy balance. In other words, they need to expend more calories than they take in. Then, once they achieve their goals, they should eat the amount of calories that they require, not more. This is energy balance.

Do You Need to Lose Weight?

If you are an endo-pear or an endo-apple, the first step is determining whether you need to lose weight. Most of us know when we're overweight; however, if you're not sure, there are several ways to determine whether you are an appropriate weight for your frame. You can calculate your body mass index (BMI) and/or your waist-to-hip ratio, or you can have your body fat percentage measured (see chapter 2 for details). If you opt for the skinfold method, I suggest that you find someone who is very experienced in using calipers and that you don't use bioelectrical impedance (the pitfalls were discussed previously). Your local university physical education program (or an experienced fitness professional at your local gym) should be able to refer you to a qualified professional who can take an accurate measurement.

Another useful guideline for women is the following calculation. Start with 100 pounds for a 5-foot-tall woman, then add 6 pounds for each inch above 5 feet (or subtract 6 pounds for each inch below). Once you have determined that number, add 10 percent to the number if you are large framed, or subtract 10 percent from the number if you are small framed.

For example, if you are a large-framed woman, 5' 5" tall, start with 100 pounds for 5 feet. Add 30 pounds for the additional 5 inches in height ($5 \times 6 = 30$). Then add an additional 10 percent for being large framed: $130 \times .10 = 13$ pounds, $130 + 13 = 143$ pounds.

With this formula, your ideal weight as a large-framed 5' 5" woman would be approximately 143 pounds.

How Many Calories Do You Need?

If you've determined that you do need to lose weight, you then need to figure out just how many calories your body requires. One way to do this is by using something known as the Harris Benedict equation.

The Harris Benedict equation provides an estimate of your basal metabolic rate, or BMR. Your BMR is the minimum level of energy required to sustain your body's vital functions. In other words, it's the amount of calories your body would require to keep all systems functioning properly if you were lying in bed asleep all day. Your BMR makes up about 60 to 70 percent of your total energy needs.

To calculate your BMR as a woman, use the following formula:

$$655 + (9.6 \times \text{weight in kilograms*}) +$$
$$(1.8 \times \text{height in centimeters}^\dagger) - (4.7 \times \text{age in years})$$

*To calculate your weight in kilograms, divide your body weight in pounds by 2.2.
†To calculate your height in centimeters, multiply the number of inches by 2.54.

Example:
Let's calculate the BMR of a 35-year-old, 140-pound woman who is 5' 5" tall.

1. First, we need to convert her weight from pounds to kilograms:

   140 pounds/2.2 = 64 kg $110/2.2 = 50$

2. Next, we need to convert her height from feet and inches to centimeters:

   5 feet, 5 inches = (5×12 inches) + 5 = 65 inches
   65 inches $\times$ 2.54 = 165 cm $66 \times 2.54 = 167.64$

3. Then, use the following formula:

$$655 + (9.6 \times 50) + (1.8 \times 167.64) -$$
$$(4.7 \times 18) = 1,352.152 \times 1.725 =$$

$$\boxed{2,332.4623}$$

$$655 + (9.6 \times \text{weight in kilograms}) +$$
$$(1.8 \times \text{height in centimeters}) - (4.7 \times \text{age in years})$$

$$655 + (9.6 \times 64 \text{ kg}) + (1.8 \times 165 \text{ cm}) - (4.7 \times 35)$$

$$655 + (614.4) + (297) - (164.5)$$

$$655 + (614.4) + 297 = 1,566.4 - 164.5 = 1,401.9$$

$$\text{BMR} = 1,402 \text{ kcals/day}$$

Once you have calculated your BMR, you'll need to determine how many additional calories over and above your BMR you would need to fuel the activities of your daily life. This will give you a good idea of what your total caloric requirements are.

Activity Factor

If you are sedentary (little or no exercise, desk job), multiply your BMR by 1.2.

If you are lightly active (light exercise/sports 1–3 days per week), multiply your BMR by 1.375.

If you are moderately active (moderate exercise/sports 3–5 days per week), multiply your BMR by 1.55.

If you take heavy exercise (hard exercise/sports 6–7 days per week), multiply your BMR by 1.725.

Going back to our example, let's assume that this woman is lightly active, so we would multiply her BMR by an activity factor of 1.375.

$$1,402 \text{ kcals} \times 1.375 = 1,927.75 \text{ kcals/day}$$

This means that according to the Harris Benedict equation, the woman in our example would need roughly 1,930 kcals/day to maintain her current weight. Or putting it another way, she needs about 530 additional calories per day to fuel her activities of daily living. Keep in mind that there is a margin of error in this calculation of about 10 percent or, in this woman's case, roughly 200 calories.

This also means that the woman in our example should never eat less than her basal metabolic rate of 1,402 calories per day, to ensure that she is eating enough to provide the basic energy required for bodily functions. If you eat fewer calories than what is required, your body will slow your metabolism down in an attempt to conserve energy and will actually sabotage your weight-loss efforts.

Calories Do Count: Weight Loss by the Numbers

So by this point, you should know whether you need to lose weight and how many calories you need to maintain your current weight. Now let's apply this information and make it work for you.

As I mentioned, ideally, it's not a good idea to lose more than half a pound to two pounds per week. Research indicates that when you lose weight faster than this, you lose lean body tissue in the process, which ironically slows down metabolism and makes it more difficult to keep weight off over time.

One pound of body fat is equal to 3,500 calories. That means you need to burn off 3,500 calories more per week (or 500 calories per day) with exercise or eat 3,500 fewer calories per week (or, again, 500 fewer calories per day). Now, trying to burn 500 calories more or eat 500 calories less per day can be a daunting task.

Consider for a moment that the 140-pound woman in our example would need to walk briskly for 1 hour and 15 minutes or run a 9-minute mile for about 40 minutes in order to burn about 500 calories. That's a lot more activity than most people do—an ambitious (and probably not realistic) goal. Likewise, trying to eat 500 fewer calories per day is also difficult.

Rather than trying to eat 500 fewer calories per day or burn 500 calories more, a better idea is to try to achieve a 500-calorie deficit per day with a combination of both. That way, it's not as overwhelming, because you need to burn only 250 more calories per day and eat 250 fewer calories per day. Therefore, if we look at the 140-pound woman in our example, she could burn 250 calories by

Walking briskly for 40 minutes

Jogging for about 20 minutes

Gardening for 50 minutes

Swimming for 30 minutes

Biking for 30 minutes

Cleaning house for about 60 minutes

Then she could cut 250 calories out of her diet by any combination of the following:

Switching from 2 tablespoons of full-fat mayonnaise to 2 tablespoons of light mayonnaise (saves 100 calories)

Using 2 tablespoons of fruit spread on her toast instead 2 tablespoons of butter (saves 100 calories)

Switching from 2 tablespoons of full-fat roquefort cheese salad dressing to reduced-calorie roquefort dressing (saves more than 100 calories)

Switching from an 8-ounce glass of whole milk to skim milk (saves about 60 calories)

Eating $1/2$ cup of rice instead of a cup (saves 100 calories)

Taking $1/2$ the bun off her hamburger (saves 100 calories)

Switching from 1 tablespoon of mayonnaise to 1 tablespoon of mustard on her sandwich (saves about 100 calories)

Switching from a grande caramel Frappuccino with whipped cream to a grande nonfat latte (saves 252 calories)

Switching from two scoops of full-fat ice cream to two scoops of fat-free frozen yogurt (saves 246 calories)

Switching from 2 tablespoons of margarine on her toast to 10 pumps of spray butter (saves 200 calories)

From these examples, it's easy to see that watching your calories doesn't necessarily mean deprivation. It's just about making little changes throughout the day. The same is true for exercise. You could break up that 40 minutes of brisk walking per day into two 20-minute segments. Try to combine physical activity with something that you need to do anyway, such as walking the dog or taking the kids to the bus stop.

If you consistently eat and burn a combination of 500 fewer calories per day, you will lose about a pound a week. In this way, you can work backward to determine how long to expect the process to take. Figure that if you are looking to lose 10 pounds, a healthy and realistic time frame would be ten weeks or two and a half months. Losing it sanely over time, you'll ensure (1) that you lose fat weight, not lean body tissue; and (2) that you don't slow down your metabolism with your efforts.

The Endos ●●●

The Commandments of Weight Loss and Control

Again, I want to empower you with the knowledge to make smart choices, all the time. That way, no matter where you are, whether it's a wedding buffet or McDonald's, you'll have strategies to stay on track and meet your goals. So, here are some can't-miss rules to help endos lose weight and stay slim.

Commandment #1: Thou shalt count thy calories.

Calories count; don't let anybody tell you differently. A recent study found that almost 80 percent of Americans believe that when it comes to weight loss, the type of food that they eat is more important than the total number of calories. Nothing could be further from the truth.

When it comes to weight loss (or weight gain, for that matter), it's all about the calories. You show me a woman who is steadily gaining weight, and I'll show you someone who's eating more calories than she is burning. Chances are, however, like most of us, she may not be aware of how many calories she really needs to eat or what specific foods in her diet are putting her over the top.

Let's take a minute to look at what a calorie actually is. *Calorie* is short for *kilocalorie*, a scientific term for a unit of energy. Calories are literally a way to measure how much fuel you would get out of a food if you were to burn it up in a special device called a bomb calorimeter. The more calories the food has in it, the longer it takes to burn up. For example, a 75-calorie apple burns up much faster than a 600-calorie piece of chocolate cake.

The same is true for burning those foods in your body. Moreover, body fat is a storage form of energy. When you eat more energy than you need, your body stores the rest as fat. Eat less than you need, and your body will tap into that fuel storage to keep you going.

Many endo-pears and endo-apples have what I call "eating amnesia." That is, they aren't fully conscious of all the calories they ingest. All calories count. I said earlier that if we cut out 250 calories per day and burn about 250 more per day with exercise, we can expect to lose about a pound a week. But it's very easy to eat those 250 calories on the fly, without even thinking about it. Just a few handfuls of M&Ms at your desk, a 16-ounce smoothie, half of the average muffin, a small serving of French fries—any one of these—and, voila, you're there.

That's why it is key for all endos who are trying to lose weight to keep track of what they eat in a food journal (as described previously). Certainly, you don't have to do it for the rest of your life, but if you do it for several weeks, you will

- Become more accountable and aware of what you really eat in the course of a day. You tend to make better choices when you know that you will be recording what you eat.

- Spot trends that undermine your progress. Are you eating too few calories in the morning so that you are ravenous in the afternoon and end up either overeating or making poor food choices?

- Learn how many calories are actually in what you eat. Be sure to read the label and check the serving size for the foods you eat because on many food packages, what's listed as a serving size is really half of what you are eating. For example, the serving size of a popular chocolate chip cookie ice cream sandwich is listed as 225 calories, but that is for half a sandwich. When was the last time you ate half of an ice cream sandwich?

- Become aware of how much you drink, and I don't necessarily mean alcohol. Many women don't realize how many calories are in the beverages they consume and how fast these can add up. Consider the calorie counts of these everyday beverages:

   An 8 oz. glass of orange juice—110 calories

   A 16 oz. hot chocolate with whipped cream—450 calories

   A 12 oz. can of soda—160 calories

   A 16 oz. fast-food milkshake—720 calories

   A piña colada—260 calories

   A margarita—170 calories

   A glass of water—zero calories!

It's very easy to cut out calories just by watching what you drink. For example, if in the course of a day you substituted

A diet soda (0 calories) for a regular soda (162 calories)—*saves 162 calories*

A whole orange (45 calories) for a glass of orange juice (110 calories)—*saves 65 calories*

A 4 oz. glass of red or white wine (80 calories) for a standard-size margarita (170 calories)—*saves 90 calories*

Total calories saved = 317 calories

That's a pretty painless way to knock out 300 calories!

Commandment #2: Watch thy portion sizes.

Again, as Americans we tend to supersize everything. Keep in mind that restaurant portions may be up to eight times larger than standard portion sizes. Here are some easy guidelines for figuring what constitutes a serving size.

One serving of meat, poultry, or fish is the size of a computer mouse or a deck of playing cards.

One serving of fruits or vegetables is about the size of your fist.

One serving of pasta is about the size of a scoop of ice cream.

One serving of cheese is the size of your thumb.

Two tablespoons of oil would fit into a shot glass.

One serving of pretzels and chips is the size of a cupped handful.

One serving of rice would fit into a cupcake wrapper!

Look at the calorie counts on food packages or on the nutrition information pamphlets that are available at major food chains. Remember that people often eat two or three times more than they think they do, so try to be honest when evaluating how many calories you take in. Always err on the side of overestimating your intake, not underestimating. If you don't, you'll only be fooling yourself and undermining your own weight-loss efforts in the long run.

Commandment #3: Thou shalt trim the fat.

The average American gets a whopping 37 percent of her daily calories from fat, and 16 percent of that fat is typically artery-clogging saturated fat. This is considerably more than the 30 percent of calories from fat (with no more than 10 percent from saturated fat) recommended by the American Heart Association. Gram for gram, fat has more than twice as many calories as carbohydrates or proteins, so fat's not just bad for your heart health, it's bad for your waistline, too.

This means that when you're watching your caloric intake, you must keep an eye on how much fat you eat. A gram of either carbohydrates or protein is only 4 calories, whereas a gram of fat is 9. This means that you can eat a lot more volume of food from carbohydrates and protein for the same number of calories. Consider, for example, that 2 table-spoons of blue cheese dressing is about 150 calories. For that same number of calories, you could have

1 6 oz. container of low-fat vanilla yogurt

3 oranges

7 hard pretzels

3 oz. of grilled skinless chicken breast

4 cups of broccoli

6 (that's right, 6) cups of low-fat microwave buttered popcorn

The fact is that lower-fat foods give you more volume for your calorie "dollar."

Also, while you're keeping your fat intake low, try to make the fats that you do eat as healthful as possible. Here's the lowdown on the best and the worst of fats:

Best Choices	Next-Best Choices	Worst Choices
olive oil	mayonnaise[†]	bacon fat
canola oil	trans fat–free margarine[†]	butter
natural peanut butter	corn oil	solid vegetable shortening
avocados	safflower oil	coconut
walnuts[*]	pumpkin seeds	cream cheese[†]
fish,[*] especially mackerel, lake trout, herring, sardines, albacore tuna, and salmon	sunflower seeds	sour cream[†]
		half and half
flaxseed oil[*]		
almonds, peanuts, pecans, and cashews		

*High in heart-healthy omega-3 fats
†When choosing these foods, opt for the low-fat or fat-free versions whenever possible.

Commandment #4: Thou shalt focus on fiber.

Foods high in fiber are a dieter's best friend because they fill you up without adding any calories. The bulk they provide can keep you fuller longer, thereby acting as a natural appetite suppressant. High-fiber foods come from plant sources, fruits, and vegetables. Fiber is literally the edible part of plants that our systems can't digest.

Not surprisingly, most folks in the United States aren't getting enough of the fiber they need. The recommendation is that we get 25 to 30 grams of fiber per day, and most of us get only about half that much.

There are actually two types of fiber: insoluble and soluble. Insoluble fiber holds onto water and adds bulk to the foods that you eat. This bulk helps push food through the GI tract faster, promoting regularity and a healthier digestive system. Good sources of insoluble fiber include wheat bran, vegetables, whole grains, and beans.

Soluble fiber, on the other hand, actually combines with water in the intestinal tract to make a gel-like substance. This gel does two important things. First, it catches cholesterol and helps remove it from the body before it ends up clogging arteries. Second, it slows down the release of sugar into the bloodstream (making a fiber-rich diet particularly important for people with diabetes). This allows insulin to work more effectively and prevents dramatic rises and falls in blood sugar levels. Soluble fiber is found in oats, oat bran, barley, and legumes.

One cautionary note: unless you enjoy spending lots of time in the bathroom, don't go "fiber crazy" all at once. When you add fiber to your diet, you need to do it slowly over a period of time. If you take in much more than you're used to, you can experience abdominal cramping, bloating, and diarrhea. A good rule of thumb is to try to add one more high-fiber food to your diet every three days or so, allowing your body to adjust. And because fiber requires water to do its job, be sure that you drink plenty of it.

Commandment #5: Thou shalt be aware of thy starches.

Complex carbohydrates (also known as starches) are the body's primary nutritional fuel source; however, it's very easy to overeat these important foods. Endo-pears and endo-apples need to be particularly aware of their portion sizes.

Consider that the average restaurant-size pasta dinner consists of 4 to

5 cups of pasta, with some popular chains serving portions as big as 8 cups. The recommended number of servings from this food group is six to eleven per day. This means that one serving of pasta could represent between eight and sixteen servings—in just one meal!

The average deli bagel may be four to five servings of carbohydrates—in a single bagel. Rice is another tricky starch. The standard portion size is equivalent to the amount that would fill a cupcake wrapper. Think how much bigger than that the rice portions are at your favorite restaurant.

Another problem with starchy foods is the toppings you put on them. Butter, margarine, cream sauces, and even olive oil will each add another 100 calories per tablespoon to the meal. A couple of teaspoons of these toppings will easily add another several hundred calories to a restaurant dinner that is already a virtual calorie bomb.

As a weight-conscious endo-pear or endo-apple, you need to be aware of (1) what constitutes a serving size, and (2) how many calories are in that serving, on average. In general, keep in mind that the portions tend to be about half as big as you'd think they'd be, and they tend to be in the 100-calorie range, give or take about 20 calories.

Here are some specific examples:

Food	Serving Size	Calories	"Real World" Serving
pasta	½ cup (cooked)	100	6 oz.—600 calories
bagel	½ of a 2 oz. bagel (very small)	90	4–5 oz. bagel—400 calories
muffin	½ of a 2 oz. muffin	100	4–6 oz. muffin—500 calories
baked potato	3–4 oz.	100	16 oz. potato—450 calories
beans	½ cup cooked	140	2 cups—560 calories
hot dog/ hamburger bun	½ bun	100	3 oz.—250 calories
cold cereal	½ cup	75	2 cups—300 calories
hot cereal	½ cup cooked	75	4 oz.—450 calories
popcorn	3 cups popped	90	7 cups—580 calories

The Bottom Line for the Endos

Let's review the five commandments that all endos should keep in mind:

Count calories.

Watch portion sizes.

Choose low-fat foods.

Eat more fiber.

Watch your starches.

There truly is no magic secret to losing weight and keeping it off. If endos just focus on obeying these five commandments and nothing else, it will be virtually impossible for them not to succeed in their weight-loss efforts.

Suggested Meal Choices for the Endo			
Breakfast	Lunch	Snack	Dinner
1 cup dry whole-grain cereal (not granola)	tossed salad with 3 oz. grilled chicken (no cheese, nuts, or croutons)	1 cup of low-fat frozen yogurt	broiled salmon with lemon
½ cup blueberries	1 tbsp. dressing		steamed mixed veggies (with dash of spray "butter")
1 cup skim milk	small multigrain roll		½ sweet potato
coffee or tea with skim milk	1 pat of butter		fresh pineapple
	apple		
¼ cup of scrambled egg substitute (Better 'n Eggs, Egg Beaters)	sandwich of small whole wheat pita with 3 oz. fresh turkey breast, mustard, lettuce, and tomato	banana with smear of peanut butter	lean hamburger patty with lettuce, tomato, and ketchup on whole wheat English muffin
whole wheat English muffin with 1 tbsp. margarine	orange		small green salad
slice of cantaloupe			1 tbsp. dressing
coffee or tea with skim milk			mixed berries with fat-free Cool Whip topping

Breakfast	Lunch	Snack	Dinner
1 cup multigrain hot cereal 1 cup skim milk ½ cup strawberries coffee or tea with skim milk	"mock pizza" (whole wheat tortilla, 1 oz. low-fat mozzarella, and 2 tbsp. marinara sauce, with steamed mushrooms, broccoli, fresh tomatoes, etc., on top) small green salad 1 tbsp. dressing slice of watermelon	1 cup of low-fat yogurt with sprinkle of dry cereal	grilled chicken and veggie stir-fry cooked in non-stick pan with spray oil (3 oz. white-meat chicken breast, broccoli, carrots, snow peas, and water chestnuts) ½ cup brown rice fresh mango

For beverages, endos should choose mostly water and sparkling water with lemon or lime, coffee or tea (up to two times per day), and not more than 1 diet soda per day.

The Mesos ●●●

The Commandments of Staying Lean and Mean

Meso-pears and meso-apples, with their naturally higher muscle tone and higher metabolism, have less of a tendency to gain weight than their endo-pear and endo-apple sisters do. Where endos are usually very efficient fat storers, mesos are less prone to store body fat and therefore have a bit more leeway with regard to their food choices and portion sizes. Mesos needn't be as concerned as their endo counterparts with counting calories. Certainly, they may gain the occasional five pounds or so, but ordinarily, to have significant weight problems, they would have to be out of control with their eating habits on a regular basis.

The following commandments are guaranteed to keep mesos the natural hard bodies that they are.

Commandment #1: Thou shalt eat close to nature.

Because mesos naturally have more lean body mass and higher metabolisms, they can usually eat more calories than an endo body type of the same size can. This doesn't give mesos the license to be junk food junkies, though. Quite the contrary, mesos need to be sure to fuel their naturally athletic frames with the most nutritious choices available.

The easiest way to do this is to focus on the nutrient density. Nutrient density means getting the most "bang for the buck" from your food. In other words, nutrient-dense foods typically have the most health benefits and the fewest calories.

How do you know what nutrient-dense food are? It's easier to spot them than you might think. Overwhelmingly, these foods are (1) close to nature and (2) vibrant in color. When making a food choice, mesos should first ask how close it is to its most natural state, and second, is it a dramatic color? These foods are fresh fruits and vegetables, lean proteins, whole-grain carbohydrates, and heart-healthy fats.

Our bodies naturally thrive on the foods that Mother Nature has provided. Again, keep in mind that processing almost never makes food better. Typically, the more processing that goes into foods, the lower the nutritional content and the higher the calorie count. One notable exception to this rule are frozen fruits and vegetables, which, when frozen right after being picked at peak freshness, will retain their vitamin and mineral content longer than will fresh fruits and veggies that are left hanging around for days in the refrigerator's crisper.

Still not sure which foods to choose? Here's a list of some nutritional powerhouses:

Vegetables	Fruits	Whole Grains	Beans/ Legumes/ Nuts and Seeds	Proteins (choose organic varieties whenever possible)	Low-Fat Dairy
broccoli	blueberries	whole wheat	soybeans	chicken	low-fat or fat-free cheese
collards/ mustard greens/ Swiss chard/ kale	apples	oats	black beans	turkey	
	bananas	brown rice	kidney beans	lean beef	
	oranges	barley	lentils	salmon	low-fat or fat-free milk
	papayas	buckwheat	walnuts	cod	

Vegetables	Fruits	Whole Grains	Beans/ Legumes/ Nuts and Seeds	Proteins (choose organic varieties when- ever possible)	Low-Fat Dairy
sweet pota- toes/yams w/skin	strawberries cantaloupe prunes	quinoa yellow corn	flaxseed almonds cashews peanuts	halibut snapper shrimp eggs	low-fat or fat-free yogurt
carrots					
beets					
avocado*					
tomatoes*					
olives*					

*Technically, these items are fruits.

It sounds simple enough, but in this world of fast foods, convenience foods, and highly processed carbohydrates, it's easy to end up consuming lots of foods with very few nutrients that are high in calories. A white-flour bagel for breakfast, an energy bar for a snack, a slice of pizza for lunch, fast food for dinner—you can see how easy it is to rack up the calories while taking in little in the way of nutrition.

Commandment #2: Thou shalt listen to thy stomach.

As human beings, we are born with an innate ability to eat as many calories as our body requires without overeating. If you have ever fed a newborn baby, you know this is true. Babies stop nursing or drinking their bottles when they feel they've had enough. They take in what they need, and then they're done. They know when they're sated, and they don't want or need any more. The same is true for young children; they eat until they are satisfied, and then they stop eating before they are overfull.

Unfortunately, most of us lose touch with this ability to self-regulate at some point in our childhood. That's a shame, because this mechanism serves people well in regulating their weight. It enables them to trust their own bodies to tell them how much they need and puts them in control of how much they eat.

Keep in mind that the human stomach is about the size of an average fist; however, it has the ability to stretch to three times its normal size!

If you overeat on a regular basis, the stomach remains more stretched out than it was before. Once your stomach gets used to this higher volume of food, you'll need more food than before to feel satisfied.

Because mesos have naturally decent metabolisms, it's easy for them to keep their weight under control if they stay in touch or get reacquainted with their natural ability to regulate their intake. This process is related to the concept of eating meditation that I mentioned in the previous chapter. Here are some tips for learning how to listen to your stomach.

1. **Eat only when you are actually hungry.** Don't practice what I call preemptive eating—in other words, (a) eating when you aren't hungry, (b) eating because you might get hungry later, or (c) eating because it's mealtime and you're supposed to eat. Take a moment and listen to your body. Are you hungry? If so, eat. If you're not, don't. There is no reason to eat just because it's mealtime, you are supposed to be eating, or other people are eating. Eat because you are hungry. Period. End of sentence.

2. **Eat before you are starving.** It's not a smart idea to wait so long to eat that you are ravenous and are likely to overeat, even if this means having a snack to hold you off so that you aren't out-of-control hungry by the time you sit down to a meal. If you're concerned that eating a snack will ruin your appetite, then ruin it with something nutritious. Choose a healthful snack that's very nutritious. So what if you can't eat as much at mealtime because of it? You're getting the nutritional benefits, and that's what's most important.

3. **Eat slowly and savor what you're eating.** Eating a meal doesn't mean setting a new speed record. What's the rush? Certainly, there are times when we really do have to wolf down a meal, but many times we don't, and yet we still consume our food much faster than necessary.

   Try taking smaller bites, pausing to chew the mouthful slowly so that you can actually taste it before you swallow. Put down the fork occasionally and take a break. Try eating at half of your normal speed. Typically, it takes about twenty minutes for your brain to get the signal from your belly that it's full. Slow down and give your body a chance to send you the signals that it's had enough.

4. Stop eating when you're full. There is no benefit to continuing to eat once you're satisfied. At that point, you are only ingesting more calories than you need and you run the risk of feeling ill. So what if there is a lot left on the plate? Your body is not a human garbage disposal! So what if it tastes good? You tasted it, you enjoyed it, and now you've had enough—so stop!

Follow these steps, and you will never feel bloated after eating a meal. More important, you'll get back in touch with your body's own regulatory system. This connection puts you in control for a lifetime of painless and easy weight management, without deprivation or guess-work.

Commandment #3: Thou shalt go for the grains.

Again, pound for pound, mesos can eat a bit more than endos can and still maintain a healthy and appropriate weight. Because the majority of your daily calories should come from the bread and cereals group, the most appropriate way for mesos to spend those "leeway" calories are on high-quality, multigrain, complex carbohydrates.

Unfortunately, since the late 1990s, with the rise in popularity of high-protein, low-carbohydrate diets, *carbohydrates* has become a dirty word. Carbs have been touted by many as the great evil associated with weight gain. Not true.

Remember that any calories eaten to excess of what the body needs will be stored as fat. This means that if fats, carbohydrates, or proteins are consumed beyond what the body needs, they can result in weight gain. There is nothing unique about the calories found in carbohy-drates. In fact, a Harvard study of 27,000 people found that middle-aged individuals who ate 40 grams or more of whole grain per day tended to be three and a half pounds lighter than those who ate less whole grain.

Carbohydrates are actually the most important of the macronutrients because, unlike fats and proteins, they are a vital fuel source for some of our most vital organs, including the kidneys, the nervous system, and the brain.

The trick here is eating the right kind of carbs. Most of the carbo-hydrates you consume should be complex carbohydrates from whole-grain sources, not simple sugars. Of the six to eleven servings of grains recommended per day, an absolute minimum of three of these servings should come from whole-grain sources. The average American, however, consumes one serving or less per day of these important whole-grain foods!

Whole grains are key because in addition to having carbohydrates, which provide energy for the body, they also have fiber, B vitamins, antioxidants, and minerals such as iron, zinc, copper, and magnesium. Good sources of whole grains include whole wheat, wild rice, brown rice, bulgar, buckwheat, oatmeal, millet, and barley.

The Bottom Line for the Mesos

Let's review the three commandments that all mesos should follow:

Focus on the nutrient density of foods.

Get in touch with your body's innate hunger mechanism.

Eat more healthful whole grains.

If mesos get back in touch with their bodies' built-in weight control system and focus on getting back to nature, they will not only maintain their weight, they will be taking a major step toward ensuring a lifetime of good health.

Suggested Meal Choices for the Meso

Breakfast	Snack	Lunch	Snack	Dinner
1 cup hot multi-grain cereal	1 cup low-fat yogurt	tossed salad with 3 oz. grilled chicken	low-fat granola bar	broiled salmon with lemon
slice of melon	piece of fresh fruit	1 tbsp. dressing		steamed mixed veggies (with dash of spray "butter")
1 slice whole wheat toast with smear of natural peanut butter		small multigrain roll		
		1 pat of butter		1/2 sweet potato
1 cup skim milk		cup of mixed berries		mixed berries with fat-free Cool Whip topping
coffee or tea with skim milk				(*continued*)

Suggested Meal Choices for the Meso (*continued*)				
Breakfast	Snack	Lunch	Snack	Dinner
2 slices of French toast made with egg substitute and whole wheat bread bit of maple syrup 1/2 cup strawberries coffee or tea with skim milk	handful of whole wheat crackers skim milk latte	sandwich of 2 slices of whole wheat bread with 3 oz. fresh lean ham, 1 slice low-fat cheese, mustard, lettuce, and tomato handful of cheese-flavored or caramel rice cakes	small cone of low-fat frozen yogurt	lean hamburger patty with lettuce, tomato, and ketchup on whole wheat English muffin small green salad 1 tbsp. dressing fresh pineapple
2 pieces of whole wheat toast with smear of natural peanut butter and sliced banana 1 cup skim milk coffee or tea with skim milk	skim milk latte apple	egg-white omelet made with egg substitute (steamed mushrooms, broccoli, fresh tomatoes, sprinkling of low-fat shredded cheese) whole wheat English muffin with 1 tbsp. margarine low-fat frozen yogurt cup of fat-free chocolate pudding with fat-free Cool Whip topping	handful of whole wheat crackers with smear of natural peanut butter	grilled chicken and veggie stir-fry cooked in nonstick pan with spray oil (3 oz. white-meat chicken breast, broccoli, carrots, snow peas, water chestnuts) 1/2 cup brown rice fresh mango

The Ectos ●●●

The Commandments of Putting (and Keeping) "Meat on the Bones"

If you're like most ectos, you're probably sick and tired of people always commenting about your weight. Perhaps they gawk at you in envy, asking how you stay so slim. Or worse yet, maybe they stare at you in horror, informing you that you look emaciated or even anorexic. Either way, it can be very annoying to have your weight always be a major topic of conversation, especially if you're trying to gain weight, not lose it. It's also interesting that as an ecto, you generally don't get a lot of sympathy from people when you tell them that you have a hard time keeping weight on. Tell folks that, and they tend to get either sarcastic or dismissive, with comments like, "Oh, you poor thing," or "I wish I had your problems."

If you are an ecto, though, you know just how frustrating it can be to always feel too scrawny, too thin—to wish you had more curves. Hopefully, you're already following the basic guidelines given in the previous chapter to ensure that you're getting the proper nutrition for good health. However, due to your fast-as-lightning metabolism, you'll need more healthful calories overall than your meso or endo sisters do. Just as it takes a reduction of 3,500 calories to lose a pound of body weight, it takes the addition of that same amount to put weight on. This means that in order to gain a pound a week, you would have to consume an extra 500 calories per day. It can be difficult for ectos to work that many extra calories into their diets. Here are some commandments that can make your struggle to gain weight a whole lot less challenging.

Commandment #1: Thou shalt eat calorically dense foods.

It's important that ectos eat foods that are not only nutrient-dense but also calorically dense. That means choosing the close-to-nature foods that pack more of a high-calorie punch. These are typically foods that, although very healthful, also contain a bit more naturally occurring sugars and fats, which racks up their calorie counts. Top choices in this category include nuts, seeds, olives, dried fruits, avocados, natural fruit juices and nectars, 1 or 2 percent milk products, olive oil, and trans-fatty-acid-free margarines. Here are a few suggestions on how to work them in easily to your present diet:

Munch on a trail mix of nuts, seeds, and yogurt-covered raisins.

Add slices of avocado and/or low-fat cheese to your salads and sandwiches.

Keep energy bars and fig bars on hand for easy on-the-go snacks.

Dip your whole-grain bread into olive oil or spread on the margarine.

Eat granola. It's healthful but provides a lot of calories per serving. Just avoid those made with coconut and coconut oils, which contain lots of saturated fat.

Feel free to let the salad dressing flow. Just use heart-healthy monounsaturated fats, such as olive and canola oil, whenever possible.

Eat homemade muffins made with olive oil or margarine, whole-grain flour, and plenty of nuts and/or raisins.

Slather natural peanut butter on your whole-grain bread.

Pour plenty of maple syrup on your buckwheat pancakes.

Commandment #2: Thou shalt guzzle thy calories.

One easy way to get the extra calories that your high-performance "ecto engine" needs is to drink them down. A beverage won't fill you up the way that solid food does and therefore allows you to take in far more calories than you normally could.

Although your faster ecto metabolism might allow you to drink endless sodas or artificially flavored drinks, you should try to avoid them as much as possible. Not only do these high-calorie beverages provide zero in the way of nutrition, they will also wreak havoc with your blood sugar levels.

Sugary beverages raise your blood sugar levels. The body then compensates by releasing the hormone insulin in an attempt to get sugar out of the bloodstream and into the cells. Once insulin shuttles sugar into your cells, your blood sugar level will dip down again. All of this happens in a very short period of time, making you feel tired and/or irritable.

Instead, choose drinks that not only taste good and have plenty of calories but also provide as much nutrition as possible. Top choices include milkshakes made with low-fat milk and frozen yogurt or fruit smoothies of yogurt, fruit, and natural fruit juices and fruit nectars. To add even more of those much-needed calories, you can toss in a packet of a nutrition supplement powder (such as Myoplex or Met Rx). These drinks can easily add 300 to 600 extra calories or more and will go a long way toward helping you pack on some pounds.

Commandment #3: Thou shalt snack often and supersize thy meals.

The bottom line for ectos is that they need to eat more than meso and endo women of the same stature do, in order to gain and maintain their weight. There's no getting around it—they need to consume more calories relative to their size than other body types do. Because of that, it's usually difficult (if not impossible) for ectos to eat as many calories as they need in just three meals. That's why ectos should aim for a minimum of six small meals per day, or three meals and three snacks, which means eating approximately every three waking hours.

The other focus for ectos is to try for modest increases in the portion sizes of everything that they eat. Portion control is not a phrase that an ecto needs to be concerned with. Foods like brown or wild rice and pasta (preferably whole wheat), which are notoriously difficult to portion control, are perfect for ectos. Also, you can sneak in even more calories by adding olive oil, low-fat cheese, and lean proteins (like shrimp or chicken) to your pasta dish and nuts and raisins to your rice pilaf.

Ectos are unique, in that their ability to rapidly burn off their food (just by breathing) gives them a free ride to indulge in anything they want. Keep in mind, however, that there is more to eating than taking in calories. Your body needs optimum nutrition to feel its best and keep you healthy. Just because you could be a junk-food junkie without gaining weight doesn't mean that you should be.

Remember that ectos are not immune to heart disease. Diets high in fat (particularly saturated fats) can block coronary arteries and cause high blood pressure. These risks are just as dangerous for slim folks as for their bulkier counterparts.

The Bottom Line for the Ectos

Let's review the three commandments that all ectos should follow:

Choose foods with high caloric and nutrient density.

Use beverage consumption to sneak in extra calories.

Eat often and heartily, aiming for at least six meals per day.

Ectos need to use their God-given right to indulge in foods wisely. It's almost like getting a big bank account that you could spend any way you wanted. Spend it wisely; don't fritter it away on things your body doesn't need. In other words, eat and enjoy, but always with an eye toward the choices that are in your body's best interest.

Suggested Meal Choices for the Ecto

Breakfast	Snack	Lunch	Snack	Dinner	Snack
French toast with whole wheat bread and whole eggs, with maple syrup and margarine	trail mix with plenty of nuts and dried fruits	sandwich of turkey breast (large multi-grain bun, low-fat cheese, lettuce and tomato, sliced avocado, and low-fat mayonnaise)	low-fat granola bar	baked salmon with bread-crumb topping	peanut butter and jelly sandwich made with natural peanut butter and fruit spread on whole wheat bread
strawberry-banana smoothie with low-fat yogurt and milk	large glass of low-fat milk	fig bars	large glass of fruit juice	veggie stir-fry made with canola oil	large glass of fruit juice
				large portion of brown rice	
				whole wheat bread with olive oil dunk	
				green salad with plenty of olive oil and vinegar	
				low-fat yogurt sprinkled with granola	

Breakfast	Snack	Lunch	Snack	Dinner	Snack
large bowl of whole-grain cereal large glass low-fat milk banana 2 slices of whole wheat toast with smear of natural peanut butter	yogurt shake walnuts and raisins	lean hamburger on large whole wheat roll, low-fat cheese, lettuce, and tomato large sweet potato with margarine veggie stir-fry with canola oil large glass of juice	energy bar	large bowl of whole wheat pasta made with olive oil, white-meat chicken, olives, and Parmesan cheese green salad with plenty of olive oil and vinegar whole wheat rolls with margarine low-fat granola bar large glass of fruit juice	string cheese crackers apple
omelet with low-fat cheese and fresh veggies cooked in margarine large glass of juice whole wheat bagel with margarine	low-fat yogurt topped with low-fat granola and nuts	whole wheat pasta with shrimp, veggies, olive oil, and Parmesan cheese whole wheat bread with olive oil large glass of juice	tortilla chips with guacamole	bean soup with crackers grilled chicken breast stir-fried veggies with olive oil brown rice pilaf with nuts and raisins	natural peanut butter and banana on whole wheat bread large glass of low-fat milk

how to embrace your shape: loving your body type

Most women spend much of their lives wanting to look like other women. Ectos want to be endos, endos want to be ectos, mesos want to be ectos. It's part of human nature to want what we haven't got. The proverbial grass truly is greener on the other side. Nowhere is this more evident than in the way women view themselves—and one another.

The more women you talk to, the easier it is to believe that nine out of ten of us are dissatisfied with the way we look. In my sixteen years in the fitness industry I have never had a female client come to me and say, "You know, I'm already pretty terrific. I'd like to work on changing a few things, but I'm really very happy with myself the way I am today." Not once.

Invariably, my first session with a client consists of a litany of all the things that she hates about her body and wants to change. And then there are the inevitable comparisons to other women whom she wants to look like. "I wish I had so-and-so's legs (or butt, arms, etc.)."

The fact of the matter is that nobody gets it all. There will always be someone with something that you could potentially envy. That's life. Life isn't fair, and we aren't all created equal. Inevitably, there will be someone who is thinner, younger, and more fit; who has bluer eyes, shinier hair . . . it goes on and on.

All of us have heard shocking stories of women going to extremes to transform themselves into someone totally different from what nature intended them to be. Women in Asia undergo multiple surgeries to have their features made more Caucasian. A Hollywood starlet submits to yet another surgery to change something about her body (that only she believes needs changing). A New York City socialite has multiple surgeries to make her features more feline. The list is endless.

While it's perfectly normal to notice other women and to appreciate their beauty, there is a real danger in longing to be something that you're not. That "Why can't I be more like her?" attitude is a very disempowering way to live, because it sets you up for a lifetime of self-loathing and frustration. Unfortunately, though, if you're like most women, you probably have this point of view to some extent.

Nearly all of us are more comfortable putting ourselves down than taking a compliment. No woman wants to be perceived as conceited. So much so, that it's practically a social obligation to comment about how much you hate your (fill in the body part) when your friend bemoans all her problem areas. "You think that's bad, look at how fat my —— is" . . . and so forth, and so on. We actually use negative self-talk as a way of bonding with our sisters. It's a kind of "we're all in the same club" mentality. "Hey, I'm just like you. I hate my body, too!"

But what if we lived in a world where we were able to make connections with other women based on feeling good about ourselves? "Hey, you're beautiful and fabulous—and so am I!"

The truth is, you have every right (and, I would argue, an obligation to yourself) to be comfortable in your own skin. That's where you live, after all. So you're not perfect—inside or out. So what? Who is? There is no reason in the world that you need to apologize for being exactly as nature made you.

Moreover, you are entitled to celebrate all those things that make you beautiful—physically, emotionally, and spiritually. Sure, I'll admit it's not an easy point of view to embrace, but once you do, it is very empowering.

I once went to a women's self-esteem workshop where we did a very interesting exercise. We broke into groups of two. Each woman had to sit facing her partner, who paid the woman one sincere compliment after another. "You have beautiful eyes." "You dress nicely." "You smell really good." And so on.

The trick was that after every compliment, you had to say out loud to your partner, "Thank you. It's true." You weren't allowed to make faces, shake your head no, or say anything else. You had to just sit there and take it. All of us found it very uncomfortable.

Afterward, the teacher said, "From now on, whenever someone pays you a compliment, I want you to say 'Thank you' out loud and then silently to yourself, 'It's true.'" I think that was great advice.

I call this avoiding compliment rejection, and it's just one simple step that all of us can take toward self-love and acceptance. Not only does it teach you to accept a compliment gracefully, it also validates the opinion of the person who paid you the compliment. Think about it. Whenever you reject someone's compliment by saying something like, "Oh, no, that's not true," it's almost like saying, "What do you know? You're an idiot." Whereas a simple, gracious "Thank you" says that you respect the other person's opinion and you appreciate the sentiment behind the comment.

It is my hope that you will use all of the tools in this book to help you take care of your body with the exercise and the nutrition that are right for your body type. As a parting gift, I would like to offer some tried-and-true methods that you can use to get on the path to greater self-acceptance and self-love.

1. *Fake it till you make it!* Imagine how much needless angst would be eliminated if every woman honestly believed: "I am exactly who I'm supposed to be. I'm already perfect in my own way, and I'm improving every day."

Try saying those sentences aloud right now. If you're like most of us, you probably don't mean it. It probably feels boastful and uncomfortable, but changes in our fundamental core beliefs have to start somewhere. One way to make those internal changes is to act "as if" or fake it till you make it. In other words, play a trick on yourself and pretend that you believe it. Go one step further and try to take on the behaviors and thoughts that you imagine you would have if you did believe it.

How would you look at yourself? What kind of internal dialogue would you have with yourself? How would you treat yourself? Your reality is largely whatever you believe it to be. You may be playing a role today, but if you do it consistently, those beliefs and behaviors will become a part of you and will cause a fundamental shift in your self-concept.

2. *Step away from the scale.* I've already outlined the ways in which women terrorize themselves with constant weigh-ins. I cannot emphasize this enough. You are not three digits on a bathroom scale! Rather than focus on a number that you haven't seen since high school but believe you should weigh, focus on your health. If you follow what is outlined for your body type in this book, the numbers will take care of themselves. Rather than jumping on the scale once a day (or more), pay attention to the fit of your clothes. You can tell if you are putting on or losing weight. If so, make the appropriate adjustments to get yourself back on track. If you absolutely must weigh yourself, however, do so no more than once per week. Do it at the same time and under the same conditions.

3. *Stop terrorizing yourself in the mirror.* I remember once reading a magazine article about a beautiful Hollywood actress. She was talking about how whenever she felt "too good" about herself, she would stand naked in front of a full-length mirror and squeeze her butt in a way that would show "all the cellulite." She said this motivated her and kept her on her diet and exercise program.

That amazed me! All I could think was (1) why does this breathtakingly beautiful woman believe she shouldn't feel "too good" about herself? (2) Why does she feel the need to motivate herself though self-hatred? and (3) If this flawless woman can find things to criticize about her looks, the rest of us are in deep doo-doo.

Yet I cannot tell you the number of women (and I myself was guilty of this for years) who feel compelled to stare at themselves in the mirror in various stages of undress and do a critical analysis of every imperfection. As women, we tend to zero in on our flaws, magnify them tenfold, and scrutinize them mercilessly. To make matters worse, most of us tend to do this after a big meal, the day before we get our periods, and/or under the most unflattering light possible.

For most of the women I know, self-disgust does nothing to motivate them to take care of themselves. Quite the contrary; having that kind of mentality makes people throw their hands up in despair and take on a "why bother" attitude.

I always tell my clients, "Whenever you look in the mirror, instead of isolating your individual blemishes and blowing them up larger than life, try to focus on the big picture instead." Remember, you are not your body parts—you are not even the sum of those body parts. You are a body, a mind, and a spirit.

How many people have you known who became more and more attractive the longer you got to know them? At some point in your relationship, you probably could no longer be objective about their looks because you developed great affection for them and saw them as a lot more than a physical presence. Keep in mind that the same is true for how others view you.

Whenever you do look at your body, try not to break it down into its elements. Look at the overall picture and think to yourself, "This is me. And I'm exactly the way I'm supposed to be." Moreover, if you aren't able to look at yourself in a full-length mirror without feeling positive (or, at the very least, neutral) thoughts about yourself, I honestly suggest getting rid of that mirror.

4. *Keep things in perspective.* If you continually measure your physical appearance against that of celebrities, you're sure to be disappointed, time and time again. The reality is that most celebrities are better looking than the general population. No surprise there! That's one reason people pay to see them—because they are pretty to look at!

Sure, it's fine to appreciate their attractiveness, but you must keep in mind that these are not normal people. They don't have normal lives. And in order for them to keep their highly unusual jobs, they need to look as close to perfect as possible.

To accomplish this, they have a team of experts and virtually unlimited financial resources at their disposal. They have personal chefs, personal trainers, trailers with gyms in them on movie sets, nannies, personal assistants, drivers, housekeepers, hairdressers, makeup artists, stylists . . . you name it. In other words, they have all the time, the resources, and the support to make sure they always look their absolute best.

In an ideal world, we wouldn't compare ourselves to other people, but, for better or worse, those evaluations are a part of human nature. Therefore, rather than comparing yourself to someone who is in the good-looks business, compare yourself to real people. Look at your family, your coworkers, and your friends. Remember what folks actually look like.

There is a great line in an episode of one of my favorite TV shows, *Sex and the City*. In it, Sarah Jessica Parker's character, Carrie Bradshaw, is in a charity fashion show, wearing a very skimpy outfit. She is nervous about how she looks and asks her friend Stanford Blatch if she looks like a model. To which he replies, "You're the modeliest of the real people." I think that says it perfectly. There are models and there are real people. Always try to see things for what they are and be realistic. Models and celebrities are genetic rarities. If we were born fortunate enough to look like Gisele, we'd be making big bucks on our looks, too.

5. Remember what fit females actually look like. The heroin-chic look of some models and actresses has nothing to do with being in good condition. That waiflike look is based on not exercising and/or not eating enough. Unless you are an ecto-apple or an ecto-pear, you were not designed to be skinny. Being underweight is not a part of being healthy.

Think of real-world examples of fit women: Gabrielle Reece, Brandi Chastain, the Williams sisters, Anna Kournikova. These women aren't thin. They are toned, they are fit looking, they are not emaciated. If female athletes were underweight, they wouldn't have the energy and the power they need to excel in their respective sports.

6. Don't join the catfight. Women can be really horrible to other women, catty and downright mean. I don't think I'm being antifeministic when I say that you could probably make a case for this having something to do with Darwinian evolution. Women who were competitive and aggressive were probably more successful at getting men and procreating, thereby creating more women who were competitive and aggressive.

Nevertheless, there is no reason to tear your fellow women down. We are all lots more alike than we think, and few things in this world are better than sisterhood.

Think about your best girlfriend growing up. How special was that bond with her? A person whom you knew was totally on your side. A person you could tell all of your secrets to and know that they'd be safe. As women, we need each other, too. We'd all do better and live in a happier world if we focused on looking out for one another, mentoring one another, and taking care of one another. The female experience is totally unique. Only another woman can truly understand what it is like to have the two X chromosomes. As women, we need to remember this.

One easy way that we can be part of a sisterhood is not to engage in critical analyses of other women's bodies. You don't benefit in the least by saying mean things about other women or staring daggers at them. Not only should you try to avoid saying and thinking negative thoughts about yourself, you should also avoid it with your sisters. Avoid offering unsolicited opinions to your friends. Don't say anything if you can't say something nice. Don't hold yourself or other flesh-and-blood females up to unrealistic airbrushed standards.

We live in a world where eating disorders are at epidemic proportions, where most of us are dissatisfied with our appearance, and where the diet industry is a $50 billion business. It's a world gone mad, where virtually every one of us feels unhappy with her appearance. It's a hostile environment in which to be a woman. We can either choose to live in this world or create one of our own choosing.

I suggest that we take a page out of the men's book when it comes to how we evaluate ourselves. Men usually don't judge themselves by what they look like but rather by their accomplishments. Haven't you seen extremely overweight men in Speedo bathing suits parading down the beach as if they were stars on *Baywatch*? Most men are okay with their bodies, imperfections and all.

Imagine if women changed their self-concept to one based on their achievements rather than on their looks. What a momentous shift in beliefs it would be for young girls to focus on being the smartest, the most athletic, or the bravest, rather than the prettiest. What do you think the effect would be on female body image and the incidence of eating disorders? How much more could we accomplish as a gender? How much further could most of us go in our careers, education, and self-development?

I wrote this book to empower you with the knowledge that you need to take care of the body type you were born with. It's my sincere hope that you'll use these tools to take care of yourself, feel good about yourself, and look your best. Always remember who you are. You are a lot more than just your physical being. Accept yourself, cherish yourself— develop yourself to your full potential.

Again, I want to thank you most sincerely for letting me be a part of this special journey. Keep me posted on your success!

Appendix

Getting Geared Up:
A Fitness Checklist

Many of my clients want to know what they need to have on hand in order to get started. Here are a few essential items that should make your workouts more comfortable and effective.

Clothing

What to wear depends mostly on which activity(ies) you engage in and the temperature in which you'll exercise, but there are certain key items that will be staples of your workout wardrobe.

A good workout bra. Whatever you do, don't wear your regular everyday bra when exercising! Worse yet, don't go without one at all, even if you are small chested.

Regular bras simply do not provide enough support when you're moving. Look for a bra that holds the breasts in place and minimizes excessive movement. Jump up and down in the dressing room to check that your breasts are supported. The bra should be snug, yet very comfortable. You should be able to move in any direction without discomfort. Pay particular attention that the elastic underneath the breastbone isn't too tight and that the shoulder straps don't dig into your skin.

Consider one in cotton, or better yet, a microfiber. Cotton breathes, which is good. Microfibers are a better alternative, though, because they keep cold and moisture out while wicking sweat away from your skin. That means they keep you drier in the warm weather and keep you from getting wet and chilled in the cold weather.

Good sneakers. "What sneakers should I buy?" is one of the most commonly asked questions. The answer is that really it depends on what you'll be doing in those sneakers. Athletic shoe technology has gotten very sophisticated in the last twenty years, and shoes are designed for the needs of each particular activity. There are road running shoes, trail running shoes, basketball sneakers, tennis sneakers, fashion sneakers, and more. Ideally, you'll want to buy the type of sneaker for the activity that you are engaging in at that time. At one point in my career as a group fitness instructor, I had high/low impact sneakers, step aerobic sneakers, funk sneakers, running sneakers, and cross trainers. Each pair was very different, and wearing the right shoe for the right class made a world of difference.

Typically, if you're using them for general fitness, then you're best off purchasing a good cross trainer. General fitness encompasses things like walking, light jogging, general gym use, group exercise classes, or doing the workouts in this book. Cross trainers are a good general purpose shoe providing cushioning, stability, and good lateral support. Lateral support is important because it prevents the unnecessary side-to-side movements that can be injurious to your knees.

Try to shop for your sneakers in the afternoon because feet tend to swell during the day. Therefore, shoes purchased in the morning may not reflect the state of your feet later in the day.

As for how much to pay, keep in mind that you don't have to pay a fortune for good athletic shoes, but you don't want to sacrifice quality for price, either. Ultimately, all of the pressures of the activity typically end up in your feet, so make sure they are well protected.

Take your time when you shop, trying on as many premium brands as possible. See what feels the best. They should be snug and supportive but not tight or restrictive. There shouldn't be any "hot spots." Don't ever buy a pair of sneakers that you plan on breaking in; this almost never works. Remember, if they aren't comfortable when you put them on, they will absolutely kill you once you start moving.

You should have about a thumb's-width of room at the end of the sneaker, and your arch should feel completely supported. Walk (or even jog) around the store. You should have an instant "ahhh" feeling when you put them on, with plenty of cushioning with each step. Another useful technique with cross trainers is grabbing the toe and the heel of the sneaker and trying to bend the two ends toward each other. Then try to wring it out like a sponge. Ideally, a cross trainer should have decent movement when bent end to end and very little movement when you try to wring it out.

Tops. You want to dress in layers that you can peel off as your body temperature rises during exercise. Many people mistakenly believe that they should get as sweaty as possible in order for their exercise to be effective. Not true. You will (and should) sweat during exercise, particularly aerobic exercise; however, you want to allow the sweat to evaporate off you as much as possible. This means avoiding fabrics that don't breathe, such as vinyl track suits, and peeling off clothing as you start to heat up.

Over your bra, you'll need to layer up, depending on the temperature. When it's very warm, it's fine in many instances to wear just a jog bra. Most of them are designed to be seen. The ones that aren't look more like typical underwear.

Cotton T-shirts are fine; however, when you sweat they tend to stay wet and cling to you. Because the body cools itself mostly through the evaporation of sweat, a wet, soggy shirt makes it more difficult for the body to cool itself off. Again, microfiber tops do a better job of helping you maintain your body temperature and stay comfortable by bringing moisture to the outside of the shirt.

If it's warmer, opt for short-sleeve or sleeveless; if it's colder, go for longer-sleeved shirts, preferably microfiber, or cotton is a reasonable alternative.

In the coldest weather you'll need a warm top layer. Ideally, you'll want to have a good microfiber jacket or a sweatshirt in fleece or heavy cotton.

Bottoms. Again, the temperature in which you'll exercise is a major factor. If it's warm out, go for running shorts or bike/compression shorts. In cooler temps, choose tights or yoga pants. Again, cotton or, ideally, microfibers are the best choices. The typical baggy sweatpants are usually too hot to exercise in once you get moving, unless it's very cold out, in which case you may want to use them as a top layer over a pair of tights.

Also, keep in mind the types of positions that you'll be getting into during the activity. Many people aren't aware that when they bend and twist, areas that they may not want on public display are often in full view of everyone around them.

Socks. Don't underestimate the importance of good athletic socks. As with sneakers, there have been numerous advances in sock technology over the last twenty years. There are several premium brands (Thor-Lo is one of my personal favorites) that give additional cushioning and added comfort and are designed to suit the needs of particular activities, such as running, walking, and tennis. While considerably more expensive than the typical bulk package of tube socks from the discount store, high-tech socks will prevent blisters, chafing, and calluses, which can cause foot pain and impair performance.

Hats and mittens. If you're exercising out of doors, hats and mittens (or gloves, if you need to move your fingers independently) are essential for keeping comfortable during your workout.

Function and fashion. While I do think it's important to feel good about how you look in your workout clothes, be sure never to sacrifice function for style when selecting clothes. Ultimately, make your choices based on optimal performance.

Other Useful Items ●●●

Tunes. Some people enjoy peace and quiet when they exercise, but for me, nothing makes a workout fly by like good music.

I think that a personal CD player or an MP3 device is a wonderful way to stay motivated during exercise. This is particularly true for cardiovascular exercise, which can be very boring. MP3 players give you endless variety by allowing you to program what is essentially your own commercial-free radio station, filled with your favorite music.

Magazines or books. Certainly, this isn't a good idea if you're on a treadmill; however, if you do your cardio on a bike, an elliptical machine, or a stairclimber, having some trashy reading on hand is a wonderful, mindless way to pass the time. Please don't use fashion magazines if you feel intimidated by the images of models, but find some light or fun reading that you can get lost in while you exercise. I say light reading because oftentimes the movement and the effort exerted during exercise may make it difficult for you to focus on anything highly technical. But if you're one of those rare types who can absorb that kind of material while bouncing around (and it motivates you to continue exercising), more power to you!

Sweat-proof sunscreen. If you exercise out of doors, it's important to protect yourself from damaging UV rays as much as possible. That said, many of the sunscreens on the market are not exercise-friendly; they can combine with sweat and run into your eyes, making them burn and water. Look for one that specifically says it's formulated to be sweat-proof.

Hair accessories. It may sound silly, but as a woman you need to figure out a strategy for keeping hair out of your face when you exercise. As you sweat, your hair can fall into your face and eyes, becoming annoying and even painful. Headbands made of absorbent materials like terry are good, especially for women with shorter hair and/or bangs, who may not be able to tie it back any other way.

Women with longer hair should also look for hair elastics without metal on them. These bands keep hair out of your way while you work out and don't damage your hair when you remove them.

An absorbent towel. Always have a towel on hand to wipe sweat off yourself or off a surface.

Water bottle. You should drink water before, during, and after a workout, so always have a bottle of water on hand. Don't count on the water fountain; you'll only drink tiny sips on each trip and will most likely not get all the hydration you need.

A Glossary of Common Fitness Terms

aerobic   Activities that rely heavily on oxygen to generate energy. Examples of aerobic activities include power walking, jogging, cycling, and swimming.

anaerobic   Activities that do not rely heavily on oxygen to generate energy. Examples of anaerobic activities include sprinting, weight training, and boxing.

blood pressure   The amount of force on the artery walls. **Systolic blood pressure** is the top number in the reading and represents the force on the artery walls during the working or pumping phase of the heart. **Diastolic blood pressure**, the bottom number, is the force on the artery walls during the resting or filling phase of the heart. High blood pressure (or hypertension) is known as "the silent killer" because it typically has no symptoms and can result in serious complications such as heart attacks and strokes.

body fat   The amount of body fat tissue expressed as a percentage of the total body weight. A certain percentage of body fat is necessary in all human beings for optimal health and wellness; however, too much body fat is associated with health problems such as type 2 diabetes, high blood pressure, and cardiovascular disease. The typical range of desirable body fat percentages for women is between 18 and 25 percent.

carbohydrates   One of the three major nutrients used as an energy source by the body. Carbohydrates can be simple or complex. Ultimately, the body breaks down carbohydrates to maintain proper blood sugar levels. Proper carbohydrate intake is essential for optimal brain function and the performance of endurance activities. Although foods like candy and baked goods are high in carbohydrates, they are largely non-nutritive (that is to say, filled with empty calories). Ideally, most of the carbohydrates in an individual's diet should come from highly nutritious sources such as whole grains, legumes, fruits, and vegetables.

The American Dietetic Association recommends that 45 to 65 percent of one's daily calories come from carbohydrates.

calorie   A layperson's term for a unit of energy. A calorie is defined as the amount of energy that it takes to heat 1 gram of water 1 degree Celsius. When we use the term *calorie* to describe how much energy is in the foods we eat, we are actually talking about what is known scientifically as a *kilocalorie*; 1,000 kilocalories are equal to one calorie.

cellulite   The orange peel–like dimpling of skin found in 85 to 98 percent of women. It is caused by ordinary body fat trapped between pockets of connective tissue below the skin. As with ordinary body fat, cellulite's appearance can be dramatically reduced (but usually not eliminated entirely) by weight loss and the toning of flaccid muscle tissue underneath the problem area.

circuit training   A series of exercises performed in a sequence from station to station, with very little rest in between.

cross training   An exercise program that involves doing several different types of activities. Cross training is beneficial for the body because it allows for the use of different muscle groups, reduces the risk of overuse injuries, and prevents boredom. A program involving walking, yoga, and resistance training would be an example of cross training.

energy bars   A convenient, fortified snack food that contains a blend of simple and complex carbohydrates, protein, fat, fiber, and vitamins and minerals. Energy bars can serve as meal replacements or can help athletes during long endurance events. There is nothing magical about energy bars; they simply provide a quick and easy source of nutrition when it's not convenient or practical to eat a regular meal.

fat   Of the three major nutrients that can be used by the body for energy, fat is the most concentrated source. Not all dietary fat is created equal. Monounsaturated fats (found in olive and canola oil) can actually lower blood cholesterol, whereas saturated fats (found in whole-milk dairy products and red meats) and polyunsaturated fats (found in margarine and baked goods) can increase blood cholesterol and the risk of heart disease and certain cancers.

glycemic index   A system of ranking carbohydrate foods according to their effects on blood sugar. In recent years, the glycemic index has been proposed as a method of weight loss. Originally developed for diabetics, it has limited value for the general population because many factors can alter the body's blood sugar response. Although foods that are low on the glycemic index do tend to be low in calories and high in nutrition and fiber, weight loss is ultimately the result of taking in fewer calories than the body expends.

HDL   An abbreviation for high-density lipoproteins, also known as good cholesterol. Experts believe that this type of cholesterol actually protects against heart disease by carrying cholesterol away from the arteries back to the liver, where it can be processed and removed from the body.

heart rate   The heart is constantly filling and pumping blood around the body. Heart rate represents the number of times that the heart goes through this process, also known as the cardiac cycle, in one minute.

interval training   A type of workout that alternates between periods of lower- and higher-intensity activity, allowing for more total work in the same amount of time. This type of program will improve both anaerobic and aerobic fitness. A walk-jog program would be an example of interval training.

kickboxing   A general term for all martial arts disciplines that are like boxing but that also use lower-body movements such as kicking and knee strikes. Some of these workouts are actually just aerobic workouts using martial arts–inspired movements, while others involve more practical self-defense techniques.

LDL   An abbreviation for low-density lipoproteins, also known as bad cholesterol. LDL in the bloodstream can clog the arteries (in a process known as atherosclerosis) that supply the heart and the brain with oxygen, resulting in a heart attack or a stroke.

muscular endurance   How long your body can sustain a contraction or how many times your muscles can perform a contraction without fatigue. Muscular endurance is developed by using lower weights and higher repetitions (usually more than twelve but less than twenty). Yoga and calisthenics are two types of muscular endurance–training activities.

muscular strength   The maximal amount of weight that your body can move at one time. This is also called the one repetition maximum or 1 RM. Muscular strength is developed by using higher weights and fewer repetitions (typically less than eight repetitions). Olympic lifting is one type of training that's designed to improve muscular strength.

pilates   A system of specific floor exercises (mat work) and/or precise movements using special equipment designed by Joseph Pilates. Pilates's work focused on movements that strengthen the core musculature, improving posture and alignment. These workouts can be effective for improving flexibility and endurance; however, they don't make people longer and leaner as frequently touted. Getting longer would mean having a change in limb length, which would require reincarnation, not exercise. Getting leaner is a function of proper diet and sufficient cardiovascular exercise to burn off excess body fat.

protein   One of three nutrients that may be used as an energy source by the body. It is not the body's preferred energy source; however, it may be used either when carbohydrate intake is insufficient or during prolonged endurance exercise, such as a marathon. Protein is essential for the maintenance and the repair of all human tissues. The Recommended Daily Allowance for protein is 10 to 15 percent of your total calories.

R.I.C.E   An acronym for the immediate first-aid steps that you can take to treat an orthopedic injury.

Rest   Stop the activity that is causing pain or that precipitated the injury at once.

Ice   Apply ice (such as a bag of ice or frozen peas covered with a wet washcloth) to the area at once to reduce swelling and decrease pain. Keep it on the affected area for 10- to 30-minute intervals for the first 48 to 78 hours following the injury.

Compression   Use a compression bandage, such as an elastic or ACE bandage to inhibit excessive blood flow to the injury. Apply it tightly enough to cause a gentle pressure to the area, but make sure the bandage is not so tight as to cut off blood flow completely. The area should still be pink and should not feel tingly.

Elevation   If at all possible, raise or prop the injured area up so that it is higher than the level of the heart. Depending on where the injury is, this may mean that you need to lie down and/or use a chair or a pillow. This will also discourage excessive blood flow and may reduce painful throbbing.

trans fatty acids   A type of fat formed when vegetable oils are made into solid fats in a process known as partial hydrogenation. Trans fat is thought to be dangerous because it behaves like saturated fat in the body, raising the level of LDL. Some studies have suggested that trans fatty acids may contribute significantly to the development of obesity, type 2 diabetes, and certain cancers.

yoga   A five-thousand-year-old system (that originated in what is now India) that includes specific spiritual beliefs, dietary practices, and physical postures, known as asanas.

In the West, we mostly think of yoga in terms of the physical postures, as a method of exercise and stress reduction. There are many different styles of yoga, but virtually all share the same physical postures, an element of breathing, and an element of concentration or mindfulness. Some of the different styles include

Hatha yoga   A general term that typically encompasses a broad range of styles but is usually more gentle and is suitable for beginners.

Vinyasa yoga   A type of yoga based on the sun salutation (a series of twelve individual postures linked together). Movements are rhythmic and flow from one posture to the next.

Ashtanga yoga   Sometimes called power yoga. Related to Vinyasa yoga, it is also based on the sun salutation but typically involves more advanced, fast-paced movements and greater athleticism.

Iyengar yoga   Sometimes called prop yoga. Iyengar is a system of yoga that focuses on attention to perfect form in each posture. Yoga blocks, ropes, and walls are used to aid beginning and inflexible students in achieving proper alignment.

Kundalini yoga   A spiritual yoga, thought by practitioners to awaken or intensify the divine life force within the human body.

Resources

Books

Motivation and Inspiration

I love books that completely alter you for the better in some way. Each of the following books, for one reason or another, had a profound effect on me. I was quite literally one person before reading each of them and someone fundamentally different afterward. Some of these books changed the way I view the world, either philosophically or practically or both. Some of them simply validated what I already believed but had never articulated, and others just gave me inner peace. I offer them to you in the hopes that you'll get just as much out of them on your own journey.

Awaken the Giant Within by Anthony Robbins, Free Press, 1992. When I was first introduced to the author by my friend Mark, I was very skeptical. Wasn't this that big guy with the toothy grin I had seen on late-night infomercials? Wasn't this some kind of weird, New Age, power-of-positive-thinking stuff? Didn't he make people do some freaky fire-walking thing? I had a totally erroneous idea of who this man was and what he taught, and I had absolutely no interest in reading his stuff.

Despite my reservations, however, my friend persuaded me to read this book. I'm glad he did, because it was truly life-altering. I recommend it to everyone I care about, because I have yet to meet someone who didn't make positive and dramatic changes in his or her life after reading it.

Tony is a life coach who gives you all the tools you need to take control of your thoughts, direct your focus, and get whatever you want out of life. My only regret is that I didn't read it sooner.

I also highly recommend his audio programs, particularly his month-long Personal Power II Program, which guides you step-by-step through his techniques. You won't believe how much you'll be able to change your life in just thirty days. www.anthonyrobbinsdc.com/html/products/products.htm

Care of the Soul: A Guide for Cultivating Depth and Sacredness in Everyday Life by Thomas Moore, Harper Paperbacks, 1994. A beautifully written book about connecting with your authentic self, embracing your individuality, and nourishing your soul on a daily basis.

Do What You Love, the Money Will Follow: Discovering Your Right Livelihood by Marsha Sinetar, Dell, 1989. This book literally changed the course of my life. Sinetar asks you to look inside yourself to identify the things that you are most passionate about and use them to create your life's work. I picked it up after spending several unfulfilling and frustrating years working in public relations and advertising. After reading it, I knew that I had to make a radical change in my life and pursue a career in fitness.

It's Not about the Bike: My Journey Back to Life by Lance Armstrong, Berkley Trade, 2001. This is the quintessential "never say die" story. Armstrong was written off by many of his doctors as a lost cause, a man with a death sentence. Yet in the face of unbelievable adversity, he always refused to give up; he was determined not only that would he live, but that he would return as a force in competitive cycling. This book reminds you that the experts don't always know everything and that nothing is impossible if you truly believe.

The Prophet by Kahlil Gibran, Knopf, 1923. This book perfectly articulated (and validated) much of what I believed to be essential truths about life. It is one of those rare books with a gem on every page that makes you say out loud, "That's so true." Gibran shares his profound insights on love, marriage, and parenthood. Perhaps that is why it has been translated into more than twenty languages.

The Miracle of Mindfulness by Thich Nhat Hanh, Beacon Press, 1999. Written by a Buddhist monk, this guide illustrates how to be fully present in your own life. Hanh reminds us that most of us are not living in the moment. We are either thinking about the future or ruminating over the past. Meanwhile, the precious moments of our lives pass us by without our consciously experiencing them. Hanh also explains the importance of (and fundamental techniques for) starting a daily meditation practice as the ultimate state of mindfulness.

Tuesdays with Morrie: An Old Man, a Young Man and Life's Greatest Lesson by Mitch Albom, Broadway, 2002. Ironically, this is a life-affirming book about an old man's impending death. The book is a true story based on the experiences of the sportswriter Mitch Albom with his terminally ill teacher, Morrie. In sharing the final weeks of Morrie's life, Mitch learns how the reality of our own mortality can help us gain clarity about what's most important in life.

When Am I Going to Be Happy?: How to Break the Emotional Bad Habits That Make You Miserable by Penelope Russianoff, Bantam, 1989. This book is essentially an owner's manual for your own mind. Dr. Russianoff helps you identify the negative and faulty thought patterns that most of us have that hold us back from experiencing all the happiness and pleasure we deserve.

Wishcraft: How to Get What You Really Want by Barbara Sher and Annie Gottlieb, Ballantine Books, 2003. We have all heard about the importance of goal setting in getting what you most want out of life. It's impossible to set goals, though, until you get in touch with what matters to you most. This book serves as a workshop for identifying your authentic self and the direction you want your life to take. It's packed with inspirational stories of people who totally reinvented themselves and set out on a path to live their dreams.

Your Erroneous Zones by Wayne W. Dyer, HarperTorch, 1993. I read this book when I was still a teenager, and I was so taken with it that I finished it in one day. Like Dr. Russianoff and Tony Robbins, Dr. Dyer gives you insight and tools into how our own negative self-talk and erroneous beliefs hold us back from having a fulfilling existence. He details how to take personal responsibility for our own thoughts and feelings, stop blaming others for things that we want to change in our lives, and take control of the direction of our lives.

Health and Fitness

As an exercise physiologist, I tend to be drawn to highly technical and/or scientific health and fitness books that would probably put most of my readers to sleep. So I wanted to list books that make exercise science and nutrition fun and accessible to the layperson. Here are some titles that I feel do an excellent job of crystalizing complex concepts into practical tips for healthful daily living.

The Fit or Fat Woman by Covert Bailey and Lea Bishop, Houghton Mifflin, 1989. This book clarifies the differences between being thin and being fit. The authors talk about the importance of focusing on body composition rather than on scale weight and provide some commonsense advice on intelligent, long-term weight loss.

The Complete Idiot's Guide to Eating Smart by Joy Bauer, Alpha, 2003. This book should be subtitled "Everything You Wanted to Know about Nutrition but Were Afraid to Ask." Written by my good friend the registered dietician Joy Bauer, it makes nutrition education easy and fun. Joy debunks many myths surrounding diet and good eating habits, showing you how easy it really is to eat properly. This book is packed with easy-to-use tips on weight loss, eating during pregnancy, vitamins and supplements, exercise, and more.

Diets Don't Work: Stop Dieting, Become Naturally Thin and Live a Diet-Free Life by Dr. Bob Schwartz, Breakthru Publishing, 2002. This book is a must-read for the diet junkie looking for her next fix. Dr. Schwartz does an excellent job of analyzing the behaviors of naturally thin people and modeling on their success. It's a straightforward, commonsense guide that cuts through the diet hype, revealing the simple truths about how and why people lose (or don't lose) weight.

Nutrition Action Newsletter. Put out by the nonprofit organization Center for Science in the Public Interest, this newsletter actually names the names and "outs" the most unhealthful food choices. CSPI's food science experts test various food products and restaurant offerings for nutritional value and taste. They offer specific suggestions, such as the best foods to buy at the supermarket and which restaurants to frequent. I particularly enjoy the "right stuff" and the "food porn" features, which introduce the best and the worst of new food products. www.cspinet.org/nah/

Useful Web Sites

Fitness Wholesale—www.fwonline.com. This company is a great resource for well-priced fitness toys and accessories. They stock everything from resistance bands and tubing to exercise balls, steps, and weights.

Collage Video—www.collagevideo.com. Workout DVDs are a great way to interject some variety into your fitness routine, and nobody carries more of them than Collage Video. Better yet, the Collage staff, many of whom are fitness professionals themselves, actually do each and every video that they carry. They categorize each workout by type, break down the content of each one, and make recommendations as to which ones they like best.

Title 9—www.title9sports.com. This clothing company named itself after the 1972 Act of Congress that ensured that high school– and college-aged women would receive equal funding in all educational opportunities—including athletics. This act resulted in a dramatic increase in the number of women participating in and excelling in sports. The catalogue and the Web site are packed with shoes and accessories for virtually any imaginable fitness activity. The staff members at Title 9 practice what they preach and guide you toward the best choices for your particular needs.

www.geralyncoopersmith.com. Shameless self-promotion alert! I want to let you know about my upcoming fitness products, and I want to know how you're doing. So please keep in touch! I feel a connection and a responsibility to all of my readers. I want to hear from you and provide you with plenty of tools and resources to help you meet your goals. Please write and tell me what you liked about this book—and even what you didn't (please be kind!). What struggles are you dealing with in this journey toward health and fitness? What other tools could I provide to assist you? Most of all, I want the joy of sharing your successes along the way!

Index

for meso-apples, 104–105
for meso-pears, 78–79
myths about, 56–60
warm-up, cool-down for, 121, 135–136
Cat/Cow (exercise), 138
celebrities
    body type examples, 40, 41
    fashion models, 14–18
    realistic expectations and, 199–200
cellulite
    compression *vs.* consistent feature, 21–22
    defined, 210
central nervous system, 55
Chest Stretch on the Door (exercise),
    137
childbirth, 20
children, self-image of, 17–18
chocolate, 153
circuit training, defined, 210
"clean plate club," 162
clothing
    average sizes of, 14, 15
    for exercise, 123, 203–207
commandments of weight loss
    for ectos, 189–193
    for endos, 175–182
    for mesos, 182–187
    See also weight loss
competitiveness, among women, 200–201
complete protein, 164
complex carbohydrates, 163, 179–180,
    186–187. *See also* carbohydrates
compression cellulite, 21–22
conscious eating strategy, 157–158
consistent feature cellulite, 21–22
cool-down exercises
    importance of, 135–136
    individual exercises, 137–143
Coopersmith, Geralyn, 1–10
Coopersmith, Jerry, 3, 6
Coopersmith, Lee, 3, 6

Corpse Pose (exercise), 141–142
crash dieting, 29, 150. *See also* dieting
cravings, 152–156, 166–167
cross training
    defined, 210
    shoes for, 204
Curl-Ups (exercise), for endo-pears, 95
curves
    body fat and, 20
    pear body type and, 41

dairy, 161
Dancing Pony Back (exercise), 132
dehydration, 150, 161. *See also* water
densitometry, 25
depression, 153–154
diastolic blood pressure, defined, 209
diet, 7, 143
    activities of daily living (ADLs) and,
        166
    beverages, 176–177, 182, 190–191
    "Big Three" classes of nutrients,
        163–164
    conscious eating for, 157–158
    dieting *vs.* healthful eating, 156–157
    food journals, 158–161
    lifestyle changes to, 36
    natural foods in, 164–166, 183–184
    occasional treats, 155–156, 166–167
    portion size and, 162–163
    See also dieting; eating plans; eating
        strategies
diet industry, 12, 145, 201
dieting, 145–146
    average starting age for, 17
    crash, 29
    healthful eating *vs.*, 156–157
    lean body tissue lost during, 29, 150,
        173
    traps of, 146–156
    See also diet

intensity of, for individual body types, 69, 71, 78, 79, 88, 96, 105, 113
journals for, 158–161
for meso-apples, 106–111
for meso-pears, 80–86
for muscular fitness, 63–66
myths about, 56–60, 63–66, 67
overindulged eating after, 146–147
realistic expectations of, 38
specificity in, 68
warm-up, importance of, 121–124
warm-up, individual exercises for, 125–134
workout customization, 53–54
See also cardiovascular exercise; flexibility training; muscular fitness; *individual names of body types*
exertion. *See* target zone, for exercise

fashion models, 14–18
fat
  defined, 210
  in diet, 161, 162, 163
  requirements, 177–178
"fat-burning zone," on exercise machines, 56–57
FEMALES (Seven Keys to fitness), 32–38
fiber, 160, 179
Figure-Four Stretch (exercise), 141
Fine Living Channel, 9
fit appearance, 200
Fit + Female Body Type Questionnaire, 47–52
fitness programs. *See* exercise
flexibility training, 67–68
  cool-down and, 136–137
  warm-up exercise and range of movement, 123–124
Flys (exercise), for endo-apples, 116
food. *See* eating plans
footwear, 203–204

"French Paradox," 162
Frog presses (exercise), for meso-pears, 85
fruits, 160. *See also* eating plans
functional exercises, 65

genetics
  flexibility and, 67
  weight and, 37–38
Gentle Can-Cans (exercise), 133
glossary of terms, 209–213
glycemic index, defined, 211
glycogen, 150. *See also* carbohydrates
grains, 160, 186–187
gung-ho workout
  defined, 69
  for ecto-apples, 96
  for ecto-pears, 71
  for endo-apples, 113
  for endo-pears, 88
  for meso-apples, 105
  for meso-pears, 78, 79
  See also individual names of body types
gynoid (female-pattern) obesity, 41

hair accessories, 207
Hamstring Stretch in Hook-Lying Position (exercise), 141
Hand Claps (exercise), 130
Harris Benedict equation, 171–173
Hatha yoga, defined, 213
hats, 206
HDL (high-density lipoproteins), defined, 211
health problems
  of "apples" *vs.* "pears," 41
  cardiovascular exercise for, 54–56
  See also eating disorders
heart disease, 55

heart rate
    defined, 211
    reserve, 62–63
    target range, 61–63
heredity. *See* genetics
hunger, 184–186
hydrostatic weighing, 25

ideal workout
    defined, 69
    for ecto-apples, 96
    for ecto-pears, 71
    for endo-apples, 113
    for endo-pears, 88
    for meso-apples, 105
    for meso-pears, 78, 79
    See also individual names of body types
image. *See* body image
incomplete protein, 164
injury. *See* safety
interval training, defined, 211
Iyengar yoga, defined, 213

joints
    flexibility of, 67–68
    warm-up exercises and, 123
journals, 158–161

kickboxing, defined, 211
kilocalories, 175
Kundalini yoga, defined, 213

lanugo, 19
Lateral Flexion (exercise)
    for endo-apples, 119
    for meso-apples, 111
LDL (low-density lipoproteins)
    defined, 211
lean body weight, "skinny" *vs.*, 28–29
"learned selfishness," 32, 35–36
left ventricle, 55

liposuction, 22. *See also* plastic surgery
Looky Looky (exercise), 128
Lower-Back lifts (exercise)
    for ecto-apples, 103
    for ecto-pears, 76
    for endo-apples, 120
    for endo-pears, 94
    for meso-apples, 111
    for meso-pears, 84
Low-Impact Side Jacks (exercise), 126
Lunge-backs (exercise), for meso-pears,
    81
Lying Down Double Knees to Chest
    (exercise), 140
Lying Down Single Knee to Chest
    (exercise), 140
Lying Leg Circles (exercise), for endo-
    pears, 90

machines, for exercise, 56–57
Marching in Place with Arm Pump
    (exercise), 125
marketing, 16
meals, frequency of, 160, 191. *See also*
    eating plans
measurement, of weight, 23–27, 170–171,
    198
"meat and potatoes" diet, 147–148
media, images in, 17–18, 43
meditation, 142–143, 158
men
    body mass index (BMI) ranges for, 27
    "meat and potatoes" diet and, 147–148
    muscular training by, 66
    perception of female body image of,
        19–20
    self-image of, 201
    waist-to-hip ratio for, 28
meso-apples, 41, 44, 45
    eating plan for, 182–187
    exercises for, 104–111

portion size, 162–163, 177, 179–180, 191

power yoga, defined, 213

"preemptive eating," 185

pregnancy, 20, 123

premenstrual syndrome (PMS), 153–154

Prevention Magazine's BodySense, 8

protein
  defined, 212
  sources of, 163–164

Psychological Sciences, 162

Pullovers (exercise)
  for ecto-apples, 101
  for ecto-pears, 74
  for endo-apples, 116
  for endo-pears, 92
  for meso-apples, 108
  for meso-pears, 82

Push-Ups (exercise)
  for ecto-apples, 100
  for ecto-pears, 73
  for endo-apples, 115
  for endo-pears, 91
  for meso-apples, 107
  for meso-pears, 81

Quimby, Sean, 9

reading, during exercise, 206

repetitions, of exercises, 65–66

reserve, heart rate, 62–63

resistance training, 34, 58, 64–66. *See also* muscular fitness

restaurant meals, 162–163, 179–180

Reverse Flys (exercise)
  for ecto-apples, 102
  for ecto-pears, 75
  for endo-apples, 118
  for endo-pears, 94
  for meso-apples, 109
  for meso-pears, 84

R.I.C.E. (Rest, Ice, Compression, Elevation), 212

Rows (exercise)
  for ecto-apples, 100
  for ecto-pears, 73
  for endo-apples, 115
  for endo-pears, 92
  for meso-apples, 107
  for meso-pears, 82

safety, 5, 60, 68, 123. *See also* individual names of exercises

saturated fats, 161, 162, 163

self-esteem exercise, 197. *See also* body image

self talk, 197–198. *See also* body image

serotonin, 153–154

Seven Keys to fitness (FEMALES), 32–38

Sex and the City, 200

Sheldon, William, 39, 40

shirts, for exercise, 205

Shoulder Rolls (exercise), 129

Side-Lying Hip Flexor/Quad Stretch (exercise), 139

Side Stretch Standing (exercise), 138

Side-to-Side Knee-Up with Pull-In (exercise), 132

Simplify Your Life (Fine Living Channel), 9

Sinetar, Marsha, 7–8

skin, cellulite and, 21–22

skinfold measurements, 25–26, 170

sleep, 37

Slo-Mo "Karate Kicks" (exercise), 133

sneakers, 203–204

socks, for exercise, 205–206

Somatype Theory, 39–41

specificity, 68

Spinks, Evan, 4–5

spot reduction, 66

Squats (exercise)
    for ecto-pears, 72
    for endo-pears, 89
Squat-Side Leg Lifts (exercise)
    for ecto-apples, 99
    for endo-apples, 114
    for meso-apples, 106
    for meso-pears, 80
Standing Cat Stretches (exercise), 130
Standing Hip Circles (exercise), 134
starches, 179–180. *See also* complex
    carbohydrates
starvation diet, 149–150
static stretching, 67, 122
Stationary Lunges (exercise), for
    endo-pears, 90
Step Together Step Touch (exercise), 126
Step-Ups (exercise)
    for ecto-apples, 98
    for ecto-pears, 72
stomach, 184–185
storage body fat, 20–21
stress-reduction techniques
    cardiovascular exercise, 55
    Corpse Pose exercise, 142–143
    eating for pleasure and, 150–151
stretching
    for cool-down, 136–137
    dynamic, 67
    static, 67, 122
Subotovsky, Johanna, 9
sun salutation (yoga), defined, 213
sunscreen, 206–207
sweating, 58
systolic blood pressure, 209

"talk test," 61
target zone, for exercise, 61–63
taste, of food, 152
Taylor, Allison, 2–3, 5
teenagers, body image of, 17–18

Teen People, 17
testosterone, 64
"Three L's," 112–113
Three Steps Forward with a Knee/Three
    Steps Back (exercise), 125
tights, for exercise, 205
time
    eating slowly and, 185–186
    "learned selfishness," 32, 34–35
    for nutritious diet, 148–149
    for workouts, 33–34, 57–58 (*See also*
        individual workout plans)
tops, for exercise, 205
Touch-Downs (exercise), for ecto-apples,
    98
towels, for exercise, 207
trans fatty acids, defined, 213
treats, in diet, 155–156, 166–167
Tricep Kickbacks (exercise), for endo-
    apples, 117
Twist and Reach (exercise), 131
Twist and Reach with Rotation (exercise),
    131

undergarments, for exercise, 203
University of Washington, 161
Up and Down (exercise), 129
U.S. Department of Health and Human
    Services, 166

Vague, Jean, 41
vegetables, 160. *See also* eating plans
Vinyasa yoga, defined, 213
vomiting. *See* bulimia

waist-to-hip ratio, 27–28
warm-down. *See* cool-down exercises
warm-up exercises
    importance of, 121–124
    individual exercises for, 125–134